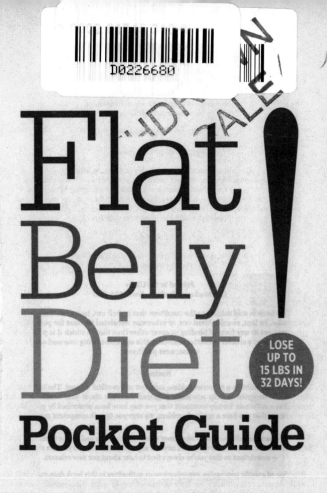

Flat Belly Diet!

LOSE UP TO 15 LBS IN 32 DAYS!

Pocket Guide

This edition first published 2011 by Rodale
an imprint of Pan Macmillan, a division of Macmillan Publishers Limited
Pan Macmillan, 20 New Wharf Road, London N1 9RR
Basingstoke and Oxford
Associated companies throughout the world
www.panmacmillan.com

ISBN 978-0-330-54440-5

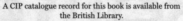

Printed in the UK by
Chatham, Kent MEs 8TD

Coventry City Council	
CEN	
3 8002 01745 310 3	
Askews & Holts	May-2011
613.25	£4.99

This book is intended as a reference volume only, not as a medical manual. The information
given here is designed to help you make informed decisions about your health. It is not
intended as a substitute for any treatment that may have been prescribed by your doctor.
If you suspect that you have a medical problem, we urge you to seek competent medical help.

Visit www.panmacmillan.com to read more about all our books and to buy them. You will
also find features, author interviews and news of any author events, and you can sign up for
e-newsletters so that you're always first to hear about our new releases.

Mention of specific companies, organizations or authorities in this book does not imply
endorsement of the publisher, nor does mention of specific companies, organizations or
authorities in the book imply that they endorse the book. Addresses, websites and telephone
numbers given in this book were correct at the time of going to press.

RODALE
LIVE YOUR WHOLE LIFE™

We inspire and enable people to improve their lives and the world around them

For more of our products visit **rodalestore.com** or call 800-848-4735

Flat Belly Diet!

LOSE UP TO 15 LBS IN 32 DAYS!

Pocket Guide

LIZ VACCARIELLO, CO-AUTHOR OF THE
NEW YORK TIMES BESTSELLING *FLAT BELLY DIET!*
WITH THE EDITORS OF Prevention.

CONTENTS

INTRODUCTION

I don't know anyone who doesn't want a flat belly. I have friends who moan about their post-baby bulge. I have colleagues who are dumbfounded by their 40-plus pooch. And I have neighbours who point guiltily to the 'beer belly' that's getting rounder, hanging lower over the belt buckle. Even my lean (lucky) friends bemoan their propensity to bloat.

When top US health magazine *Prevention* polled its readers about the body part they most wanted to change, an incredible 67 per cent said their belly. It's clear we're craving a solution to belly fat. And no wonder. Countless public health authorities continue to remind us that belly fat is the most dangerous fat you can have on your body. Even small excess amounts of it can increase your risk of high blood pressure, heart disease, diabetes, dementia and breast cancer. The combination of these two factors (health first, vanity second) is why I wanted to write the *Flat Belly Diet!* **I wanted to find the absolute best way to permanently lose belly fat.**

But I didn't just want to construct a diet and name it the *Flat Belly Diet*. I had always heard it was impossible to spot reduce, but then *Prevention*'s nutrition director came into my office with some exciting new research that showed there was a way to eat that might affect the belly specifically! The study was published in the US journal *Diabetes Care*, and it showed that eating a diet high in monounsaturated fatty acids – or MUFAs (pronounced MOO-fahs) – could help prevent the accumulation of belly fat, or more specifically, the visceral fat that we've been told to be so concerned about. MUFAs are found in foods like nuts, seeds, avocados and olive oil, and this is the only diet that features a precise serving of these healthy, filling foods in every meal you eat.

On the *Flat Belly Diet*, you'll begin with the 4-Day Anti-Bloat Jump-start. This part of the diet will leave you, on average, 2kg (4lb) lighter and at least 1 inch smaller around the waist, not to mention more confident and motivated! It's a very prescriptive phase of the *Flat Belly Diet* that enables you to flush out excess fluid. The success you will achieve during this short time frame will spark your commitment to the entire programme. The regular eating plan lasts a minimum of 28 days. This is where MUFAs take centre stage, and it's where the real fat loss begins. Each meal and each snack features a MUFA-rich food such as crunchy nuts, creamy avocado or flavourful dark chocolate.

The positive response to the *Flat Belly Diet* has exceeded my wildest expectations. I've heard from literally thousands of *Flat Belly Diet*ers thanking us for this plan. We followed nine of them in our test panel. One woman, Mary Anne Speshok, lost 7kg (15lb) and 10 inches in just 32 days – and loved the food so much she continued the plan to lose a total of 25kg (49lb) in 5 months! Although not everyone will see the same results, each of our testers was thrilled to see their bellies shrink – and, in many cases, their blood pressure and cholesterol numbers improve as well.

Still, there's nothing like scientific proof to go along with real-world success, so in the summer of 2008, we commissioned the scientists at Yale University–Griffin Hospital to study the 28-day plan's effect on visceral fat. This independent study consisted of nine female participants, all overweight or obese at the start. Scientists weighed them, measured their waistlines, took their blood and ran a battery of baseline tests to determine starting levels of cholesterol, inflammation and other important health markers. Then each woman was put through an MRI scan, so the researchers could get an internal view of her belly fat.

After 28 days on the *Flat Belly Diet*, the women were fully screened again, and the results, my friends, astounded us.

In this small but significant study, the *Flat Belly Diet* reduced visceral fat – the dangerous belly fat – by an average of 33 per cent in just 4 weeks. It also improved nearly every major health marker, lowering total cholesterol by an average of 21 points and reducing biomarkers for insulin resistance and inflammation. Participants lost, on average, 3.8kg (8.4lb) and 1.6 inches off the waist. Said David L. Katz, MD, director of the Yale Prevention Research Center, who helped oversee the research, 'If the plan were sustained, these women would be at reduced risk for heart disease, diabetes, cancer, you name it. Basically, the diet kicked butt – or, perhaps more appropriately in this case, belly!'

With this Pocket Guide, the *Flat Belly Diet* is easier to follow than ever. In letters and e-mails, you've asked for more Quick-and-Easy Meal solutions and more guidance on how to stick with the *Flat Belly Diet* when you're on the go. I enlisted the help of Tracy Gensler, MS, RD, and Samina Riaz, RD, to put together a straightforward sample eating plan for the 4-Day Anti-Bloat Jumpstart and the full 28 days of the *Flat Belly Diet*. Their meals are balanced, fast, tasty, economical and effortless to create.

With Your Ultimate 28-Day Eating Plan, plus tools to make smart eating choices wherever you are, this Pocket Guide is our answer to your questions about how to make the *Flat Belly Diet* a permanent, portable part of your life. I'm thrilled to make this diet accessible to people like you, busy people who care about their health and want the most simple and the most realistic plan. I like to think of this Pocket Guide as the no-brainer *Flat Belly Diet!* If you're eating the *Flat Belly* way already, this guide will help you continue to get results. If you aren't, here's an easy way to try it out.

Now, let's get ready to lose that belly fat!

1.

HOW TO USE
THIS GUIDE

If you've read the *Flat Belly Diet!*, you already know how easy the plan is. Just follow three simple rules and you're well on your way to a trimmer tummy, right? But if, like most women we know, you're juggling work, family and a myriad of other responsibilities, even that can sometimes be a challenge. Enter the *Flat Belly Diet! Pocket Guide*.

You don't even need to read through this whole book to get started. Just flip straight to the section that interests you now. If you want a quick overview, Chapter 2, The *Flat Belly Diet* at a Glance, gives you a summary of the plan.

If you want to try the 4-Day Anti-Bloat Jumpstart, start with Chapter 3. The jumpstart isn't necessary to burn belly fat – since it contains no recommended amount of MUFAs – but most people have found that it really helps them get in the habit of eating four meals a day, every 4 hours. Plus, of course, they love that it helps them drop weight almost instantly!

If you want to learn how to create your own *Flat Belly Diet* meals, Chapter 4 offers a MUFA Meal Maker Guide that explains how to assemble quick and tasty meals with the right ratio of MUFAs to other foods. With tips on how to shop for, store and use MUFAs and other building blocks of the diet (such as lean protein, dairy, fruits and vegetables and whole grains), this chapter gives you all the tools you need to understand how this diet works.

If you want to head straight to the supermarket to get started (you don't even need to stop and figure out your shopping list, since we've done that for you!), Chapter 5 lays out Your Ultimate 28-Day Eating Plan and takes the guesswork out of the question *What do I eat next*? We carefully designed the meal plan and grocery lists to make the most of your money – no wasted leftover portions of foods you'd love to eat but can't. We've also chosen to feature a variety of belly-shrinking MUFAs. All of the meals take less than 20 minutes to prepare, and each is filling and delicious. Plus, most of the meals are portable, so you can easily take them with you if you're on the go.

If you want to customize the 28-day eating plan to better suit your tastes, you'll find 30 additional Quick-and-Easy Meals and Snack Packs in Chapter 6 – simply substitute one meal for any other on the plan when you want a little variety.

If you're at home, our *Flat Belly Diet* Store Cupboard (in Chapter 4) and *Flat Belly Diet*-Friendly Products (in Chapter 7) will help you whip up meals quickly.

If you're concerned about how to stick to the plan when you're travelling, dining out or just running errands, we've got you covered with our Restaurant Rescue (in Chapter 7) in the airport, at the cinema or anywhere else you may go.

You'll also find quick reference lists with serving sizes and calorie counts at the end of the book to make it easy for you to calculate how much of each type of food you need for each meal. Use our quick conversion chart to decode nutrition labels and measure your servings. And throughout the book, you'll find fast, healthy eating tips and answers to questions about how to adapt the diet to special needs and tastes.

As you can see, I've designed this guide to give you just the basics so that you can make the *Flat Belly Diet* work for you. Keep this powerful little book on hand to provide instant answers about what to eat when you're at the supermarket, out with friends or anywhere else. Now it's time to get started!

2.
THE FLAT
BELLY DIET
AT A GLANCE

Prevention readers know a good diet from a fad. They tell me month after month that they like simple instructions, strategies inspired by science and plans that make logical sense. Most importantly, they want a diet that will make them healthy and infuse them with energy. That's why I made sure the *Flat Belly Diet* was designed by a registered dietitian with more than 15 years of experience helping people change their bodies and their lives with food. Any diet that contains fewer calories than you're used to eating will help you lose weight, but few weight-loss diets actually teach you how to eat to lose weight *and* maximize your health for life. Here's what makes the *Flat Belly Diet* different.

○ **It's packed with healthy foods.** I've heard that 'the hottest thing in Hollywood' is a diet that's composed almost entirely of maple syrup, cayenne pepper and lemon juice. Does this sound healthy to you? The *Flat Belly Diet* is loaded with foods you know are good for you: vegetables, fruits, whole grains, lean proteins – and of course the all-healthy MUFAs. It's the combination of these foods that makes the *Flat Belly Diet* so tremendously beneficial to your health and well-being.

○ **It's calorie controlled, not low calorie.** A registered dietitian designed the *Flat Belly Diet* to provide approximately 1,600 calories a day (which is the amount the average woman over the age of 40 needs to maintain a healthy weight), so it's by no means a starvation diet. Even better, the plan is divided into four meals per day, and you're required to eat every 4 hours. Each meal provides about 400 calories, and I guarantee you will be pleasantly surprised by how much food this actually is. (Some of the original testers never got used to how filling the breakfasts were!) By spacing out your eating times, you ensure that you never feel hungry. Ever.

○ **It's delicious!** Get ready for 'diet food' that you will actually look forward to eating. Peanut butter? Guacamole? Chocolate? Weight loss? Yes indeed. Simply said, you will love the MUFA-rich meals! I have had hundreds of letters from satisfied *Flat Belly Diet*ers thanking us for giving them a way to eat that embraces their favourite foods.

○ **It's refreshingly easy.** Since every meal is nutritionally well balanced and provides roughly the same number of calories, it's simple to substitute meals. Plus, we provide the calorie count for every component of the meal, so swapping individual foods is a no-brainer.

A lot of people who read about the *Flat Belly Diet* try to make up their own version of the plan. They might think that adding a dash of olive oil here or a slice of avocado there will somehow magically make them slim. Incorporating these healthy foods even when you're not trying to lose weight is a smart idea, but remember that MUFAs are calorie dense. If you want to lose belly fat, you must follow the *Flat Belly Diet* rules.

RULE #1: STICK TO 400 CALORIES PER MEAL.

Every *Flat Belly Diet* meal and snack contains a MUFA-rich food plus other wholesome foods to total about 400 calories per meal. It's not necessary to make sure every meal is exactly 400 calories, but it is important that, over the course of a day, you get about 1,600 calories. If one meal is a bit over 400, make the next a bit under 400 and so on.

RULE #2: NEVER GO MORE THAN 4 HOURS WITHOUT EATING.

I don't have to tell you that a diet won't work if it makes you feel hungry or tired. That's why on the *Flat Belly Diet* I ask that you eat every 4 hours. This should help you feel fuelled and energized, prevent you from feeling hungry, hold cravings at bay and keep your metabolism revved up, energized and burning calories throughout the day.

RULE #3: EAT A MUFA AT EVERY MEAL.

Monounsaturated fatty acids, or MUFAs, are the healthy oils found in many plant foods. They are delicious and packed with nutrients, and they fill you up fast (and keep you full longer). You'll find one full MUFA serving in each meal or snack of Your Ultimate 28-Day Eating Plan (page 47). Learn the five categories of MUFAs:

1. Oils

2. Nuts and seeds

3. Avocados

4. Olives

5. Dark chocolate

Later in this guide, you'll get acquainted with the full MUFA list (Your MUFA Serving Chart, page 116) and find out ways to use the MUFAs (How to Shop for, Store and Use MUFAs, page 24).

The foundation of the *Flat Belly Diet* is the Mediterranean style of eating, the gold standard of nutrition for optimal health and disease prevention. That's why the food lists are limited to whole foods or very minimally processed foods that are naturally rich in plant-based anti-oxidants, fibre and other healthy nutrients. MUFAs serve 'double duty' so to speak. They fight belly fat (as well as heart disease, type 2 diabetes, high blood pressure and cancer), and their antioxidants and other natural substances (such as resveratrol in nuts and dark chocolate, oleocanthal in olive oil, beta-sitosterol in avocado, etc.) protect your health in other ways, too!

The *Flat Belly Diet* is made up of two parts – the 4-Day Anti-Bloat Jumpstart and Your Ultimate 28-Day Eating Plan. The 4-day jumpstart is specifically designed to target belly bloat and water retention, whereas the 28-day plan featuring MUFA-rich foods is designed to help reduce belly and overall body fat.

3.

THE 4-DAY ANTI-BLOAT JUMPSTART

The goal of the jumpstart is to help you reduce or eliminate bloating and the sluggishness that accompanies it. It's important to keep in mind that the results of the jumpstart are highly dependent on your habits before you started. But many *Flat Belly Diet*ers reported feeling energized after the jumpstart and found it a great transition (physically and mentally) to the regular plan.

THE FOUR BAD GUYS OF BLOAT

Here are four lifestyle factors that can influence how prone you are to bloating or fluid retention.

1. **Stress.** A stressful event triggers hormone fluctuations that raise blood pressure and divert blood to your extremities, causing your digestive system to slow down. This can leave that last meal sitting around in your intestine a little longer, causing bloat.

2. **Lack of fluid.** It's true that you need about 8 glasses of water a day. Drinking water and eating 'watery' foods such as greens, melon and other fruits and vegetables guard against water retention and constipation, which can cause bloating.

3. **Lack of sleep.** Your nervous system depends on adequate sleep. Too little sleep disrupts the intricate workings of this system, which controls the rhythmic contractions of your GI tract and helps keep things humming along.

4. **Air travel.** The average plane maintains cabin pressure equal to 5,000 to 8,000 feet above sea level in order to provide a comfortable atmosphere for the passengers. At that altitude, free air in the body cavities tends to expand by around 25 per cent. Pressure changes also increase the production of gases in your digestive system. As the

WHERE'S THE MUFA?

Since the jumpstart attacks belly bloat and water retention, the foods selected during these 4 days are chosen based on their ability to prevent or reduce bloating. In other words, any foods you see that serve as MUFAs during the regular plan, such as olive oil, are only included during the jumpstart for their ability to help with bloating. There is not a *'MUFA at every meal'* during the jumpstart phase.

pressure in the cabin drops, the air in your intestines expands, causing bloating and discomfort. Cabin pressurization is also responsible for increased water retention because it impacts your body's natural fluid balance. Add in the dehydration caused by recirculated air, and those bloat miles add up. Before and during your flight, drink as much water as possible and walk around as often as possible during the flight.

JUMPSTART BASICS

Follow the 4-Day meal plan exactly.

This includes four smaller meals, one of which is a refreshing, bloat-blasting smoothie. You'll notice that there are generally healthy foods, such as raw vegetables and citrus fruits, that we ask you to avoid during the 4-day jumpstart. These foods provide great nutritional value, but can contribute to bloat because of their bulk and acidity. So, while we don't want you to shun these foods forever (in fact, you'll see many of them appear in your 28-day eating plan), we've banned them from your diet for these 4 days to focus on reducing your belly bloat. Instead, we carefully chose foods that deliver a lot of nutritional and bloat-free value for money *and* that need no added salt or condiments to taste good, so you won't be tempted to reach for potential bloat promoters.

THE RIGHT WAY TO HYDRATE

Limit water intake to a little over 2 litres, or up to 10 (240ml/8fl oz) glasses, per day. Your kidneys do a good job of filtering excess water, but more than this is generally not needed for non-active hours. You'll see that this is the amount of Sassy Water we ask you to drink each day during the 4-day jumpstart. We encourage you to keep that up during the 28-day eating plan, as well.

That being said, if there are foods on the 4-day jumpstart that you're allergic to, we have provided a list of approved substitutes. Again, please stick to these substitutes, which were carefully chosen to give you balanced nutrition without promoting bloat.

Eat four 300-calorie meals a day.

The 4-day jumpstart includes fewer calories – about 1,200 daily – than you'll be eating on the rest of the *Flat Belly Diet*, which allows about 1,600 per day. Eating less for these 4 days reduces the amount of food in your GI tract at any one time, cuts back on the release of stomach acids and gets your body used to a four-meal-a-day schedule.

Drink one full recipe of Sassy Water each day.

The ingredients in Sassy Water aren't just for flavour: the ginger helps calm and soothe your GI tract. Even more importantly, the simple act of making this Sassy Water every day will serve as a reminder during the jumpstart that life is a little bit different and things are going to change.

SASSY WATER

2 litres water (about 3½ pints)
1 teaspoon freshly grated ginger
1 medium cucumber, peeled and thinly sliced
1 medium lemon, thinly sliced
12 small mint leaves

Combine all ingredients in a large jug and let flavours blend overnight. Drink the entire jug by the end of each day.

Eat slowly.

When you eat quickly, you take in large gulps of air, which get trapped in your digestive system and cause bloating.

Avoid the following foods.

The following foods are off-limits for the 4 days of the jumpstart:

- Alcohol, coffee, tea, hot cocoa and acidic fruit juices
- Bulky raw foods
- Carbonated drinks
- Chewing gum
- Excess carbs
- Fatty foods
- Fried foods
- Gassy foods, including broccoli, Brussels sprouts, cabbage, cauliflower, citrus fruits, beans and pulses, onions and peppers
- Salt, from the salt shaker, salt-based seasonings and highly processed foods
- Spicy foods, including foods seasoned with barbecue sauce, black pepper, chilli peppers, chilli powder, cloves, garlic, horseradish, hot sauce, ketchup, mustard, nutmeg, onions, passata or vinegar
- Sugar alcohols, such as xylitol and maltitol, which are often found in low-calorie, low-carb or sugar-free products such as sweets, chewing gum, ice cream and jam

I CAN'T MAKE A SMOOTHIE AT WORK

The afternoon smoothie presents a challenge for many working men and women. If that's you, I recommend that you pack the ingredients separately, such as 125g (4½oz) blueberries, 240ml (8fl oz) skimmed milk, and — instead of the flaxseed (linseed) oil — 2 tablespoons sunflower seeds. Mix them in a bowl or cup. If you choose to do this, get 285g (10oz) fresh instead of frozen blueberries, leave the flaxseed oil off your shopping list, and buy an additional 70g (2½oz) sunflower seeds.

YOUR 4-DAY SHOPPING LIST

PRODUCE

- 4 medium lemons
- 230g (8oz) fresh or frozen green beans
- 285g (10oz) baby carrots
- 4 medium cucumbers
- 115g (4oz) button mushrooms
- 460g (16½oz) cherry tomatoes
- 2 bunches fresh mint

DAIRY

- 2 litres (3½ pints) skimmed milk
- 1 packet light string cheese*

FROZEN FOOD

- 285g (10oz) frozen unsweetened blueberries

DRY GOODS

- 375g (13oz) box unsweetened cornflakes
- 240ml (8fl oz) cold-pressed organic flaxseed (linseed) oil
- 240ml (8fl oz) bottle extra virgin olive oil
- 2 packets (approx 230g/8oz) roasted or raw unsalted sunflower seeds
- 450g (16oz) jar unsweetened apple sauce
- 230g (8oz) tin pineapple chunks in juice
- 170g (6oz) unsweetened raisins
- 375g (13oz) box Oats So Simple®, original variety
- 200g (7oz) can cooking spray
- 400g (14oz) brown rice

SPICES

- 1–2 knuckles fresh ginger

MEAT/SEAFOOD

- 250g (9oz) boneless, skinless chicken breast
- 230g (8oz) packet organic roast turkey slices, low-sodium**
- 340g (11oz) white fish
- 180g (6oz) tinned tuna chunks in water

ANY OF THESE APPROVED SALT-FREE SEASONINGS

If you want to add flavour to your food, use some of these *Flat Belly Diet*–approved salt-free seasonings and herbs with your meals:

- Any salt-free seasoning blends
- Fresh or dried: basil, bay leaf, cinnamon, curry powder, dill, ginger, lemon or lime juice, marjoram, mint, oregano, paprika, rosemary, sage, tarragon or thyme

*We call for light or low-fat string cheese because it is lower in saturated fat and calories. If you have trouble finding light or low-fat string cheese, though, feel free to substitute with standard string cheese.

**Organic deli meat is generally lower in sodium and fat. If your only option is to purchase non-organic meat, look for low-sodium choices.

SUBSTITUTIONS ON THE JUMPSTART

Because the 4-day jumpstart targets belly bloat and water retention, it is the most limited portion of the *Flat Belly Diet*. We encourage you to follow the meal plan exactly, but if you are allergic to one of these foods or have special dietary needs, use one of these jumpstart-approved substitutes instead. Note that all of the foods in each row are interchangeable with each other. Simply match the exact amounts mentioned here and swap away.

JUMPSTART MENU ITEM	JUMPSTART-APPROVED SUBSTITUTE
PRODUCE	
460g (16½oz) cherry tomatoes 230g (8oz) steamed green beans 115g (4oz) sautéed button mushrooms 115g (4oz) steamed baby carrots	115g (4oz) sautéed squash
DAIRY	
240ml (8fl oz) skimmed milk	240ml (8fl oz) plain unsweetened soya milk (dairy-free, vegan) 240ml (8fl oz) plain enriched rice milk (dairy-free, vegan) 240ml (8fl oz) almond milk (vegan) 240ml (8fl oz) skimmed lactose-free milk
1 light string cheese	30g (1oz) vegan cheese slices 30g (1oz) soya cheese slices
FROZEN FOOD	
115g (4oz) frozen unsweetened blueberries 115g (4oz) pineapple chunks in juice	115g (4oz) frozen unsweetened strawberries 115g (4oz) frozen unsweetened peaches

JUMPSTART MENU ITEM	JUMPSTART-APPROVED SUBSTITUTE
DRY GOODS	
30g (1oz) unsweetened cornflakes 1 packet Oats So Simple®, original variety	30g (1oz) unsweetened puffed rice cereal 30g (1oz) unsweetened gluten-free puffed rice cereal 30g (1oz) unsweetened gluten-free cornflakes
1 tbsp cold-pressed organic flaxseed (linseed) oil	1 tbsp rapeseed oil 1 tbsp walnut oil ½ tbsp pumpkin seeds 2 tbsp sunflower seeds
30g (1oz) roasted or raw unsalted sunflower seeds	30g (1oz) unsalted pumpkin seeds
60g (2oz) unsweetened apple sauce 2 tbsp unsweetened raisins	115g (4oz) tinned pineapple chunks in natural juice
110g (3½oz) cooked brown rice	115g (4oz) roasted red potatoes
MEAT/SEAFOOD	
115g (4oz) low-sodium organic roast turkey slices 90g (3oz) tinned tuna chunks in water 115g (4oz) grilled white fish 90g (3oz) grilled chicken breast	115g (4oz) gluten-free turkey slices 115g (4oz) vegetarian meat slices 1 vegetarian burger 1 vegetarian sausage

Note: In your jumpstart dinners, you are allowed only 1 teaspoon olive oil, which you can use in any way you like to help cook and flavour your foods; in other words, either you can use it to cook your vegetables or meat, or you can drizzle it over them. For other cooking, use the cooking spray.

DAY 1

THE 4-DAY ANTI-BLOAT JUMPSTART MENU

BREAKFAST

30g (1oz) unsweetened cornflakes

240ml (8fl oz) skimmed milk

30g (1oz) roasted or raw unsalted sunflower seeds

115g (4oz) unsweetened apple sauce

Glass of Sassy Water

LUNCH

115g (4oz) organic roast turkey

230g (8oz) fresh cherry tomatoes

1 light string cheese

Glass of Sassy Water

SNACK

Blueberry Smoothie: Blend 240ml (8fl oz) skimmed milk and 115g (4oz) frozen unsweetened blueberries in a blender for 1 minute. Transfer to a glass and stir in 1 tbsp cold-pressed organic flaxseed (linseed) oil, or serve with 2 tbsp sunflower seeds.

DINNER

115g (4oz) grilled white fish, drizzled with 1 tsp olive oil

115g (4oz) steamed green beans

110g (3½oz) cooked brown rice

Glass of Sassy Water

DAY 2

THE 4-DAY
ANTI-BLOAT JUMPSTART MENU

BREAKFAST

1 sachet Oats So Simple®, original variety

240ml (8fl oz) skimmed milk

30g (1oz) roasted or raw unsalted sunflower seeds

2 tbsp unsweetened raisins

Glass of Sassy Water

LUNCH

90g (3oz) tinned tuna chunks in water, drained

115g (4oz) steamed baby carrots

1 light string cheese

Glass of Sassy Water

SNACK

Pineapple Smoothie: Blend 240ml (8fl oz) skimmed milk, 115g (4oz) tinned pineapple chunks in juice and a handful of ice in a blender for 1 minute. Transfer to a glass and stir in 1 tbsp cold-pressed organic flaxseed (linseed) oil, or serve with 2 tbsp sunflower seeds.

DINNER

90g (3oz) grilled chicken breast, drizzled with 1 tsp olive oil

115g (4oz) button mushrooms, sautéed in cooking spray, if desired

110g (3½oz) cooked brown rice

Glass of Sassy Water

DAY 3

THE 4-DAY ANTI-BLOAT JUMPSTART MENU

BREAKFAST

30g (1oz) unsweetened cornflakes

240ml (8fl oz) skimmed milk

30g (1oz) roasted or raw unsalted sunflower seeds

2 tbsp unsweetened raisins

Glass of Sassy Water

LUNCH

115g (4oz) organic roast turkey

115g (4oz) steamed baby carrots

1 light string cheese

Glass of Sassy Water

SNACK

Blueberry Smoothie: Blend 240ml (8fl oz) skimmed milk and 115g (4oz) frozen unsweetened blueberries in a blender for 1 minute. Transfer to a glass and stir in 1 tbsp cold-pressed organic flaxseed (linseed) oil, or serve with 2 tbsp sunflower seeds.

DINNER

115g (4oz) grilled white fish, drizzled with 1 tsp olive oil

115g (4oz) button mushrooms, sautéed in cooking spray, if desired

110g (3½oz) cooked brown rice

Glass of Sassy Water

DAY 4

THE 4-DAY ANTI-BLOAT JUMPSTART MENU

BREAKFAST

1 sachet Oats So Simple®, original variety

240ml (8fl oz) skimmed milk

30g (1oz) roasted or raw unsalted sunflower seeds

115g (4oz) unsweetened apple sauce

Glass of Sassy Water

LUNCH

90g (3oz) tinned tuna chunks in water, drained

230g (8oz) fresh cherry tomatoes

1 light string cheese

Glass of Sassy Water

SNACK

Pineapple Smoothie: Blend 240ml (8fl oz) skimmed milk, 115g (4oz) tinned pineapple chunks in juice and a handful of ice in a blender for 1 minute. Transfer to a glass and stir in 1 tbsp cold-pressed organic flaxseed (linseed) oil, or serve with 2 tbsp sunflower seeds.

DINNER

90g (3oz) grilled chicken breast, drizzled with 1 tsp olive oil

115g (4oz) steamed green beans

110g (3½oz) cooked brown rice

Glass of Sassy Water

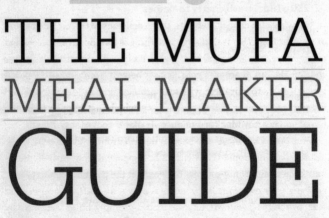

THE MUFA
MEAL MAKER
GUIDE

As we noted in the Introduction, Your Ultimate 28-Day Eating Plan in Chapter 5 is designed to give you a balanced variety of foods with plenty of MUFA-rich foods to flatten your belly, ward off disease and keep you satisfied and healthy. But you probably don't want to eat the same meals for the rest of your life! Not to worry. The choices for

MUFA-packed, delicious meals are limitless. In this section, we give you the guidelines we followed in creating the *Flat Belly Diet* meals so that you can create your own if you choose, using all your favourite foods and fat-blasting MUFAs such as oils, nuts and seeds, avocados, olives and dark chocolate.

THE BUILDING BLOCKS OF A *FLAT BELLY DIET* MEAL

As you might recall from Chapter 2: The *Flat Belly Diet* at a Glance, there are three simple rules you need to keep in mind on the diet:

Rule #1: Stick to 400 calories per meal.

Rule #2: Never go more than 4 hours without eating.

Rule #3: Eat a MUFA at every meal.

So, what else can you eat with those delicious MUFAs? The beauty of the *Flat Belly Diet* is that almost nothing is forbidden, so you can eat all your favourite foods and be as creative as you like in putting together your meals. But in order to get the most benefit from your MUFA-rich foods, it helps to pair them with lean proteins, low-fat dairy, fruits and vegetables, starches and whole grains – which just happen to be the basis for a healthy Mediterranean-style diet.

Flat Belly Diet meals are balanced, with around 35 per cent of the calories coming from MUFA-rich fats, 45 per cent from carbohydrates and 20 per cent from proteins. But don't let the percentages scare you; creating your own *Flat Belly* meals is easy – no maths required! You start by selecting your MUFA, and then you simply 'build' your meal by adding lean proteins, whole grains or fruit and (for lunch or dinner) vegetables. Refer to Your MUFA Serving Chart on page 116 for the full list of MUFAs you can choose from.

Here's how to build a *Flat Belly Diet* meal. Visual cues are provided in brackets.

If your chosen MUFA is oil, nuts or seeds, pair it with:

- 90g (3oz) lean protein (about the size of a deck of cards)
- 90g (3oz) cooked whole grain, such as brown or wild rice *or* 1 whole grain bread serving, such as half of a wholemeal pitta, *or* 125g (4½oz) fruit (1 tennis ball)
- 300g (10½oz) raw or steamed veggies (2 tennis balls)

Example: 90g (3oz) grilled salmon served over 90g (3oz) whole-wheat couscous mixed with 2 tbsp toasted pine nuts. Serve with 300g (10½oz) steamed mixed vegetables.

If your chosen MUFA is avocado or olives, pair it with:

- 90g (3oz) lean protein (deck of cards) *or* 60g (2oz) lean protein and 1 dairy, such as 1 slice cheese or 30g (1oz) grated or crumbled cheese
- 300g (10½oz) raw or steamed veggies (2 tennis balls)
- 150g (5½oz) starchy vegetables, such as beans, sweetcorn, peas or potatoes, *or* 90g (3oz) cooked whole grain *or* 1 whole grain bread serving, such as half of a wholemeal pitta or tortilla or 1 slice wholemeal bread

Example: 1 slice toasted wholemeal bread topped with 30g (1oz) sliced avocado and 90g (3oz) roasted chicken. Serve with 300g (10½oz) steamed broccoli with a spritz of fresh lemon.

If your chosen MUFA is dark chocolate, such as 45g (1½oz) dark chocolate chips, pair it with:

- 115g (4oz) fruit
- 230g (8oz) dairy, such as fat-free cottage cheese or fat-free plain yogurt *or* 170g (6oz) fat-free flavoured yogurt *or* 60g (2oz) whole grain, such as oatmeal, *or* 2 wholewheat pancakes

Example: Melt 45g (1½oz) dark chocolate chips and drizzle over 125g (4½oz) sliced strawberries. Serve with 230g (8oz) fat-free plain yogurt.

In addition to Your MUFA Serving Chart on page 116, you'll find two quick reference lists at the end of the book – Eat These Foods Regularly on page 118 and Eat These Foods Sparingly on page 128 – with appropriate serving sizes and calorie counts for all of your meal

FOOD LABEL KNOW-HOW

The Nutrition Facts labels on packaged foods can help you make *Flat Belly Diet*-friendly choices in the supermarket. Here's what to keep your eye on:

Serving Size: It's important to make the serving size one of the first things you check on the label so that you know exactly what's in the pack; use the 'Servings Per Container' to double-check the amount. So if you have a container of ice cream listing 'Servings Per Container: 4', and you plan to eat the entire container, you should multiply the calories (and everything else) by four.

Saturated Fat: The *Flat Belly Diet* saturated fat limit is no more than 3 to 4 grams per 400-calorie meal. Saturated fat content can vary considerably from brand to brand, so read labels and always select packaged products with little or no saturated fat listed on the label.

Trans Fat: Trans fat should be avoided on the *Flat Belly Diet*.

Look for products with 0 grams of trans fat listed on the label. Also check the ingredients list for the trans fat key words *hydrogenated, partially hydrogenated* and *shortening*. Labels may not add 'trans fat' to the ingredients list so it's important to know the alternative names.

Sodium: The *Flat Belly Diet* works best when you keep your total sodium below 2,300 milligrams a day. Because sodium content can vary considerably from brand to brand, it's important to read labels and to always select the lower-sodium product.

MUFA-Rich Ingredients: Since MUFAs usually aren't listed on the food label, the best way to spot them in packaged foods is to look at the ingredients lists. Look for MUFA-packed foods like oils, nuts, beans and pulses (edamame and peanuts) and seeds, avocados, olives and dark chocolate.

building blocks so that it's easy for you to calculate the amount of food you need for each meal.

Note: Foods that include a MUFA in the ingredients are not considered a MUFA for the purposes of building a *Flat Belly Diet* meal. Stick with the MUFAs (and their respective serving sizes) in Your MUFA Serving Chart on page 116 for the MUFA component of your meal.

We also give you a chart of Common Conversions on page 115 to make it easy to measure your servings and help you stay within your 400-calorie limit per meal.

HOW TO SHOP FOR, STORE AND USE MUFAS

The more you know about your MUFAs, the easier it is to make the *Flat Belly Diet* work for you! To get the most MUFA for your money, use the following tips and tricks for shopping, storing and using MUFA-rich foods, including oils, nuts, seeds, avocados, olives and our favourite MUFA: dark chocolate.

MEASURING YOUR MUFAS

Dieters who guesstimate the amounts they eat of calorie-dense MUFA-rich foods are making a big *Flat Belly Diet* no-no, since overestimating can seriously delay progress. For example, if you drizzle 2 tablespoons of olive oil over your salad (instead of the proper 1 tablespoon MUFA allowance), you'll get around 120 extra calories. Yikes. Research shows that most people underestimate serving sizes when they don't measure ingredients, so get in the habit of measuring not only your MUFAs but all of your *Flat Belly Diet* food. This will help you control not only your portions but also your hunger, to give you the health and weight loss results you're after.

MUFA #1: Oils

Plant-based oils are an important part of your *Flat Belly Diet*. Low in saturated fat and packed with good-for-you MUFAs, they're a delicious way to up your MUFA intake.

Shopping and Storing: Because all MUFA-rich oils are sensitive to heat, light and air and will go rancid if exposed to these elements or kept too long, it's important to buy in small amounts (only what you will use within a couple of months) and store properly. Select expeller-pressed or cold-pressed oils whenever possible, and store them in a cool, dark place in the back of your cupboard or in the refrigerator. Although some, like olive oil, will thicken when chilled, this does no harm to the oils, and they will resume liquid form when they return to room temperature.

Using: From robust and hearty to fragile and delicate, MUFA oils can be included in your diet in a variety of tasty ways.

- **Olive oil.** Drizzle extra virgin olive oil on salads, veggies and finished dishes, including pasta and grilled meats and fish. It's made from higher-quality, more freshly picked olives through a process that does not involve chemicals, so its fruity flavour and beneficial nutrients are uncompromised. Try using less-expensive olive oils for cooking with moderate heat (sautéing or roasting below 190°C/375°F/gas 5; medium on the hob).

- **Rapeseed oil.** Versatile and neutral flavoured, rapeseed oil is perfect for cooking that requires moderately high heat (up to about 220°C/435°F/gas 7), including baking.

- **Refined peanut oil.** With a high heat tolerance (up to about 230°C/450°F/gas 8) and neutral flavour, this oil is ideal for sautéing or roasting at high temperatures and grilling over direct heat.

- **Sesame oil.** This strongly flavoured oil adds an intense taste to marinades, dipping sauces, dressings and stir-fries.

- **High-oleic safflower and sunflower oils.** Look for natural, unrefined safflower and sunflower oils that specify 'high-oleic' on the

A MUFA MUST: PESTO

Pesto – a sauce made with olive oil, herbs, garlic, Parmesan and pine nuts – is a MUFA must-have. You can make your own or you can buy it already prepared. Keep in mind that pesto is packed not only with flavour but also with calories (around 50 to 80 calories per tablespoon), and a little goes a long way. Mix a tablespoon or two with pasta, spread some on a sandwich or spoon it over grilled fish or chicken for a MUFA-dense delicious meal.

label. This means the oils are made from plants bred to have much higher MUFA concentrations than regular safflower and sunflower oils. These mild-tasting oils won't congeal when chilled, making them ideal for dressing cold dishes like pasta salads.

○ **Walnut oil.** Strongly flavoured and heat resistant, this pricey oil is best used as a flavouring agent for special dishes.

○ **Flaxseed (linseed) oil.** Fragile and nutty-flavoured flaxseed oil has stellar nutritional benefits, but those properties are lost when the oil is heated, so it is not suited for cooking. Select cold-pressed oil, keep it refrigerated and try swirling it into a cold soup or vegetable dip, adding it to smoothies or drizzling over a salad of delicate greens.

MUFA #2: Nuts and Seeds

Packed with protein, flavour and (of course!) MUFAs, nuts, beans and pulses and seeds are practical and portable sources of MUFAs.

NUTS

Shopping and Storing

UNSHELLED: Buying nuts whole, with their natural protective covering intact, not only ensures freshness but is also much more economical than buying shelled nuts. Whole nuts can be stored in a cool, dark place for 2 to 3 months.

SHELLED: Shelled nuts (no cracking required) are sold in the baking and snack aisles of the supermarket, as well as in wholefood and speciality organic food shops, where you'll find a larger variety and better quality of nuts. Select unsalted nuts, raw or roasted without oil. Store them in airtight containers in the refrigerator for up to 3 to 4 months or well wrapped in the freezer for up to a year.

Using: Convenient and portable, nuts are a perfect on-the-go MUFA. Toss them into your handbag, suitcase or gym bag for an any-time snack or meal addition. As you'll see in Your MUFA Serving Chart (on page 116), the serving size for most nuts is 2 tablespoons; you may want to measure that amount into small zip-top plastic bags – or simply carry a tablespoon with you. Nuts are a crunchy and MUFA-rich way to jazz up just about any dish.

- **Almonds.** Whether dry roasted, raw, sliced, blanched, flaked or chopped, this versatile nut can be tossed into vegetable salads, granolas and mueslis, fruit salads and grain-based salads. Almonds can also be used in baking, ground to top or encrust fish fillets or chicken breasts, or puréed with herbs for a pesto alternative.

- **Brazil nuts.** These large tree nuts have a mild flavour and rich, coconut-like texture, and they can be coarsely chopped and mixed with rice pilaf or grain-based salads (such as quinoa, bulgur or brown rice).

- **Cashews.** With a deep flavour and creamy texture, these nuts are perfectly paired with fruit, salads, stir-fries and curried dishes.

- **Hazelnuts.** Their sweet flavour makes them especially suited for baked goods and sweet dishes. Also try them added to granolas and mueslis, fruit salads, pilafs, grain-based salads and spinach salads.

○ **Macadamia nuts.** These buttery, decadent-tasting nuts pair brilliantly with tropical fruits like pineapple, kiwi fruit and mango and with mild-flavoured fish, including halibut, sole, pollack and cod.

○ **Pecans.** With a rich, sweet flavour and a classic crunch, these nuts are a natural not only with desserts but also with spinach salads, rich puréed soups, roasted squash, baked apples and crisp-tender vegetables. Also try them stirred into pancake or muffin batter.

○ **Pine nuts.** These nut-like seeds are best puréed in pesto, toasted and tossed into salads and pasta dishes, stirred into grain dishes or mixed with sautéed greens like spinach, kale or chard.

○ **Pistachios.** These crunchy nuts are delicious mixed in savoury dishes like pasta, chicken salads and grain dishes.

TOASTY AND TASTY

Toasting nuts releases their natural oils, which not only enhances the aroma and flavour but also makes their texture crunchier. Toasting nuts at home is easier than you think. Here's how.

In the oven: Preheat the oven to 180°C/350°F/gas 4. Spread shelled nuts on a baking sheet and bake for 1 to 2 minutes. Shake the pan and continue to bake for 1 to 2 minutes longer or until the nuts start to turn light brown. Immediately remove from the oven.

On the hob: Place shelled nuts in a heavy frying pan on the hob. Heat the frying pan slowly over medium heat (shaking the pan continuously), until the nuts start to turn light brown – 2 to 4 minutes. Remove from the heat immediately.

Keep in mind that toasting nuts is a process that starts slowly, but ends quickly. Burning makes nuts taste bitter, so be sure to remove them from the heat as soon as they start to turn colour. They will continue to cook as they cool.

A MUFA MUST: NUT BUTTERS

Tried-and-true peanut butter is a MUFA-packed superstar, but to mix things up, why not try nut butters like almond and cashew? No matter what nut butter you use, be sure to buy all-natural brands in order to avoid emulsifiers and other unhealthy additives. Look for nut butters whose ingredients list shows just nuts and maybe a little salt, oil or a touch of sugar or honey.

○ **Walnuts.** With a longer shelf life (9 to 12 months in the refrigerator) than many other nuts, they make a good staple nut to stock in the kitchen. Use them crumbled onto salads, pasta and soups; puréed into a hummus-like dip; or tossed with rolled oats.

BEANS AND PULSES

Not all beans and pulses (plants that bear fruit in the form of a pod that opens along two seams) are good sources of MUFAs. Some, such as green beans, peas and lentils, are fantastic sources of protein and other nutrients, so you should definitely include them in your diet, but they don't contain MUFAs. Edamame (green soya beans) and peanuts, however, are MUFA-packed exceptions.

EDAMAME

Shopping and Storing: While fresh soya beans (deep green fuzzy pods) are sometimes available at local farmers' markets, frozen edamame are almost always available at large supermarkets. You can get them shelled and cooked, whole and cooked or whole and uncooked.

Using

UNSHELLED: The outside pods aren't edible, but eating your edamame straight from pod to mouth is a fun (and authentically Japanese) way to enjoy these beans. Just hold the pod lengthways near your lips and pinch its outer edge to press the beans against the inner seam, which will split so the beans pop into your mouth. 450g (16oz) unshelled edamame is equivalent to 230g (8oz) shelled (which is 1 MUFA serving).

SHELLED: Shelled and cooked soya beans are a perfect complement to whole grains, meats, salads, soups and vegetable dishes. They team up especially well with Asian-inspired meals.

PEANUTS

Shopping and Storing: You can choose from whole or shelled; skin-on or blanched; raw, dry roasted or boiled. Like tree nuts, whole unshelled peanuts can be stored in a cool, dark place for 2 to 3 months, and shelled peanuts can be stored in airtight containers in the refrigerator for up to 3 to 4 months or wrapped in the freezer for up to a year.

Using: Whether whole, halved, chopped, roasted or raw, peanuts can be included in stir-fries, salads, whole grain dishes and wholewheat noodle salads. They can also be used in dressings, dips and baked goods.

SEEDS

Shopping and Storing: As with nuts, you will find a larger and fresher selection of seeds in wholefood and speciality organic food shops. Whole seeds should be kept in airtight containers in the refrigerator and taste best if they are consumed within a couple of months. Once ground, seeds go bad very quickly, sometimes within a few days.

A MUFA MUST: TAHINI

Tahini, a Middle Eastern store cupboard staple, is a creamy paste made from ground sesame seeds. It's available roasted or plain in the ethnic food section of most supermarkets. It's also an ingredient in spreads and hummus (any flavour). Try it as a dip for veggies, a spread for sandwiches and a dressing for salads when mixed with oil, vinegar or lemon juice, parsley and garlic.

A MUFA MUST: GUACAMOLE

Guacamole is a dip made with ripe avocados mashed with tomatoes, onion, coriander, jalapeño chilli peppers and lime juice. You can whip up your own (see recipe on page 59) or look for supermarket brands that list real avocados as the first ingredient. Use it as a dip, in burritos or as an interesting sandwich topping.

Using: Snack on them or use whole toasted seeds sprinkled on cereal, yogurt and fruit; tossed into green salads; stirred into tuna, chicken or turkey salad; or added to savoury baked goods. Raw kernels can be sprinkled over breads and muffins before baking and sautéed with vegetables, and ground seeds can be folded into veggie or turkey burger mix or used as a base for sauces and dips.

MUFA #3: Avocados

This super-creamy fruit is not only packed with MUFAs but is also high in cancer-fighting carotenoids. It's a decidedly decadent and healthy way to get a MUFA in every meal.

Shopping and Storing: The most common avocado variety available from supermarkets is the Hass – with pebbled green skin that turns dark brown as the fruit ripens. When shopping, buying unripe or just barely ripe ensures the best flavour and texture. Pick fruits that are quite firm or give only ever so slightly to a gentle squeeze. Ripening at room temperature usually takes just a day or two (no more than three or four at most), and putting the fruit in a brown bag can speed the ripening process by about a day. Once ripe, refrigerate and use within a day or two.

Using: Spread it like butter on bread, sandwiches and burgers; mash it into dips; and use it sliced or chopped in salads and wraps.

Avocados pair particularly well with Mexican-themed dishes like quesadillas, taco salads and fajitas.

MUFA #4: Olives

These Mediterranean gems are not only chock-full of MUFAs but also rich in vitamin E, an antioxidant that protects cell membranes and reduces inflammation. From green, black or brown to Spanish, Greek and Californian, there are plenty of ways to incorporate olives into your life.

Shopping and Storing: Olives are found all over the supermarket – look for them in the condiment/pickle aisle, the wholefoods section, the deli and the international department. For the best flavour and texture, whenever possible select unpasteurized fresh olives over pasteurized jarred varieties and choose whole olives over pitted. They can be kept in airtight containers at room temperature, but they'll last longer when stored in the refrigerator.

Using: Whole, pitted or sliced olives are a wonderful snack and a tangy addition to salads, stewed chicken and meat dishes and pasta sauces.

MUFA #5: Dark Chocolate

A diet that encourages you to eat chocolate? Fantastic! Dark chocolate is a rich source of MUFAs and, if consumed in (ahem) reasonable

A MUFA MUST: TAPENADE

Traditional tapenade is a delightful mix of chopped olives, olive oil and seasonings. Used as a spread, sauce or condiment, it's easy to prepare your own (see recipe on page 181 of the *Flat Belly Diet! Cookbook*) and even easier to pick up packaged tapenade in the supermarket. Beware of artichoke, aubergine and other tapenade impostors; instead opt for olive tapenades that list olives as the main ingredient and have around 40 calories per tablespoon.

WATCH WHAT YOU DRINK

From fizzy drinks, lattes and sports drinks to juice, milk and smoothies, calories are hiding in your drinks. And don't forget about alcoholic drinks. At 7 calories per gram, alcohol delivers more calories than protein and carbohydrates, making wine, beer and cocktails nutrient-poor calorie traps. In fact, one large margarita can easily contain as many (or more) calories as an entire meal.

Studies show that the calories from liquid drinks don't satisfy your hunger as well as the calories from solid foods and have little or no effect on how much you eat over the course of the day. On the *Flat Belly Diet,* stick with thirst quenchers that won't throw off your weight loss efforts. Water, coffee and tea are good picks – and of course a *Flat Belly Diet* fave, Sassy Water (see page 11 for recipe).

quantities, a healthy and enjoyable component of the *Flat Belly Diet*.

Shopping and Storing: You can buy your dark chocolate in chunks, bars or chips. Look for chocolate with at least 60 per cent cocoa solids, and keep in mind that heat affects flavour and consistency, so your favourite eating chocolate may not be the best performer as a baking chocolate. Chocolate should be stored in its original wrapping in a cool, dry place (but not in the fridge, which is too cold and moist) and away from strong-smelling items (chocolate absorbs odours). Stored properly, most dark chocolate will last up to a year.

Using: Dark chocolate is divine all on its own, of course, but it can also be swirled into breakfast oats; mixed into muffin and pancake batter; sprinkled into yogurt; and eaten with fruit.

WHAT ELSE CAN I EAT?

In addition to a delicious 'MUFA at every meal', your *Flat Belly Diet* is packed with lots of other hearty and wholesome foods that will keep you feeling satisfied and hunger-free. As we noted earlier, there are no forbidden foods on the *Flat Belly Diet*, but you do want your meals to be a balanced mix of MUFA-rich fats; good-for-you carbohydrates, including whole grains, fruits and vegetables; and lean proteins, like fish, chicken, beans and low-fat dairy. This combination of foods, eaten at regular intervals (every 4 hours), will keep you burning belly fat, while maintaining energy, muscle mass and bone density.

Here are a few general guidelines to keep in mind to help you eat and lose weight the *Flat Belly Diet* way.

Guideline #1: Consume no more than 4 grams of saturated fat per meal.

Saturated fat raises levels of LDL ('bad' cholesterol) in your blood and, in turn, increases your risk of cardiovascular disease and stroke. Animal products, like meat and dairy products, are the main sources of saturated fat, but tropical oils – coconut oil and palm (or palm kernel) oil – and cocoa butter are also high in saturated fat. Small amounts of saturated fat are also found in some other plant foods, including MUFA-rich olive oil and nuts, so it's impossible to eliminate the saturated fats altogether. However, you can greatly decrease the amount in your diet by

THE 'FAT' FACTS OF DARK CHOCOLATE

With the limit on saturated fats, you might be wondering why dark chocolate is included in the *Flat Belly Diet* plan, since the amount we recommend (45g/1½oz of chocolate chips or the equivalent) contains quite a bit more than 3 grams of saturated fat. There are different types of saturated fat, and the type in dark chocolate (stearic acid) largely gets converted in the body to oleic acid, which is a MUFA! So although dark chocolate has a higher saturated fat content – and when you include it in one of your *Flat Belly Diet* meals, your total saturated fat will be over the 4-gram max – this type does not tend to raise blood cholesterol levels and is considered heart healthy.

substituting healthier fats, like olive oil and rapeseed oil, for straight saturated fats like butter. In Your Ultimate 28-Day Eating Plan, we've kept the saturated fat level as low as possible (around 3 grams per meal), so you see it *is* possible to have flavour without saturated fats!

Guideline #2: Ban trans fat.

Like saturated fat, trans fat increases levels of LDL ('bad' cholesterol) in your blood. But that's not all. Trans fat also lowers levels of HDL ('good' cholesterol), which helps keep blood vessels clear, making trans fat a really bad fat. Trans fat is produced when hydrogen is added to liquid oils to make them solid (and extend their shelf life), and it is found mostly in packaged products. Labels may not add 'trans fat' to the ingredients list so it's important to know the alternative names. Look for the words *hydrogenated, partially hydrogenated* and *shortening*. If you spot these terms in the list, put that food down and keep looking!

Guideline #3: Avoid artificial sweeteners, flavourings and preservatives.

Aspartame is one of the most prevalent artificial sweeteners used in foods and drinks today. It's found in diet drinks, sugar-free yogurts and puddings, chewable vitamins, gum and even high-fibre cereal. But ever since the FSA approved it in 1982, many nutrition researchers have disputed its safety and many people have complained that it causes headaches, dizziness and mood changes. Artificial food colourings used in some sugary cereals and sweets have been linked to hyperactivity and behavioural problems since the 1970s. Nitrates, which add flavour (mostly to meats), have been linked to various types of cancer. And these are just a few of the many artificial additives in our food. Try to avoid artificial anything (colours, flavours, preservatives); instead pick whole foods as often as possible and look for foods with ingredients you can easily recognize and pronounce. The *Flat Belly Diet*-Friendly Products list (page 105) can also help you identify additive-free packaged foods.

Guideline #4: Limit sodium to less than 2,300 milligrams a day.

Sodium causes water retention (which not only makes your weight temporarily spike on the scale but also causes unsightly puffiness) and increases your risk for high blood pressure, which can lead to

BE SAVVY ABOUT SODIUM

Keeping your *Flat Belly Diet* sodium below 2,300 milligrams per day is simple. Here's how:

Limit salty MUFAs. While most MUFAs are low in sodium, olives are indisputably salty, so it's best to limit olives (and olive dishes) to no more than once a day. Also read the labels carefully on packaged MUFA-rich foods like olive-based tapenade, pesto and nut butters, and always pick the lower-sodium products.

Ditch the shaker. Put away the salt shaker and use the following *Flat Belly Diet*-approved (sodium-free) seasonings instead: fresh or dried basil, dill, ginger, marjoram, mint, oregano, rosemary, sage, tarragon and thyme as well as aged balsamic vinegar (use lightly: 1 tablespoon = 5 calories), bay leaf, cinnamon, curry powder, lemon or lime juice,

paprika and salt-free seasoning blends.

Go whole. The *Flat Belly Diet* encourages you to limit highly processed foods (they are the main source of excessive sodium in the average diet) and instead to use real foods made from whole ingredients like fruits, vegetables, whole grains and lean proteins.

Read labels. When you do purchase packaged foods (like bread, tinned beans, sauces and MUFA-rich nut butters and tapenade), always compare brands. Sodium content can vary considerably from brand to brand, so read labels and always select the lower-sodium product. And be sure to rinse tinned beans, vegetables and tuna in a colander under cool running water for 2 to 3 minutes to remove up to 30 per cent of the sodium.

heart and kidney disease, as well as stroke. Because the *Flat Belly Diet* is about flattening your belly *and* enhancing good health, the *Flat Belly Diet* recommends keeping your total sodium below 2,300 milligrams a day (or approximately 575 milligrams per meal).

HOW TO SHOP FOR, STORE AND USE THE OTHER MEAL BUILDING BLOCKS

The *Flat Belly Diet* is packed with a variety of delicious and good-for-you foods that, when combined with MUFAs, offer a healthy way to unload belly fat. And the more you know about these nourishing food picks, the more likely you are to embrace this healthy way of eating for a lifetime. To help you get the most out of your *Flat Belly Diet*, use the following tips and tricks for shopping, storing and using the other *Flat Belly Diet*-friendly foods, including lean proteins, dairy, fruits and vegetables and whole grains.

Proteins

For good health and weight loss and to keep the saturated fat in your meals within the *Flat Belly* limit of 3 to 4 grams, it's important to always make your protein picks *lean* picks.

BEEF, POULTRY AND PORK

Shopping and Storing: While beef, poultry and pork are packed with lots of high-quality protein, if your picks aren't 'lean', they can also pack your arteries with a hefty dose of saturated fat. Here's what to look for in the supermarket.

- **Beef:** Pick the leanest cuts, including steaks and roasts (topside, silverside), fillet, sirloin and chuck steak.
- **Poultry:** Pick skinless chicken or turkey parts. Boneless, skinless turkey and chicken breasts are the leanest picks.

- **Pork:** Select the leanest cuts, including pork loin, fillet and ham.

- **Minced meat:** Select 90 per cent or higher 'lean' mince and low-fat minced turkey breast or chicken.

- **Cold cuts:** Select lean turkey, chicken, turkey ham or ham. Uncured or preservative-free versions are your best picks.

- **Vegetarian meat substitutes:** Look for veggie burgers, mince, etc., with no more than 2 grams of saturated fat (no trans fat) and 480 milligrams of sodium per serving.

Keep in mind that Nutrition Facts labels on fresh meat and poultry are not compulsory, so for even more help making your best picks, simply ask your butcher for nutrition information (most supermarkets carry in-store Nutrition Facts). The colour of fresh meat is highly unstable and therefore is not the best indicator of freshness. Instead, pay attention to the smell (fresh, not sour) and the feel (firm, not mushy) of the meat. Also, check use-by and sell-by dates and buy the product with the latest date.

Fresh cuts of beef, poultry and pork can be stored in the refrigerator

SHOULD I BUY ORGANIC MEAT?

Organic poultry and meat are good choices if you are concerned about antibiotic use and pesticides. Organic meat (marked 'Soil Association Organic Standard' with a white circle) doesn't contain residual pesticides, because the animals must be given pesticide-free organic feed or must graze on land on which pesticides haven't been used for at least 3 years.

The animals also can't be given antibiotics nor can they be fed animal by-products. Also, organic meat tends to be lower in sodium and fat and packaged organic deli meat often lasts longer. For this reason, you'll see that Your Ultimate 28-Day Eating Plan calls for organic meats. If you choose to purchase non-organic meat, please look for low-sodium choices.

for 2 to 3 days after the sell-by date and in the freezer for 6 to 12 months. Minced meat can be stored in the freezer only up to 3 months. Try freezing individual pieces of meat or burger patties. They thaw more quickly, and you can pull out one or more depending on your needs, making preparation a snap.

Using: You can roast, braise, grill or bake your lean cut of meat and use it in a variety of healthy and tasty ways. Use it in a sandwich, toss it into a salad, pair it with pasta, mix it in grain dishes or serve it all on its own. You can also check out the plethora of delicious MUFA-rich, lean meat recipes featured in the *Flat Belly Diet! Cookbook*.

FISH

Shopping and Storing: Fish is a *Flat Belly Diet* protein-superstar. Loaded with heart-healthy omega-3 fats, it's a high-quality protein source that is low in saturated fat and full of healthy nutrients. Here are a few things to keep in mind.

- When selecting seafood, fatty dark fish (such as salmon and tuna) provide a good source of the omega-3 fats. Light-coloured fish (such as snapper and sole) as well as a variety of shellfish are good choices, too. They're low in fat but high in protein.

- If possible, pick wild, sustainable fish over farmed fish (farmed fish have higher levels of contaminants than those caught in the wild), but keep in mind that farmed fish is better than no fish at all.

- Breaded or seasoned frozen fish should have no more than 3 grams of saturated fat (0 grams of trans fat) and 480 milligrams of sodium per 115g (4oz) fillet or serving or 90g (3oz) cake.

- Buy fish tinned in water (not oil), and the lower the sodium, the better. You can also get tuna or salmon in a convenient (no draining needed) vacuum-packed pouch from some shops.

○ When buying whole fish, look for moist skin; bright red, moist gills; firm flesh that bounces back when touched and clear eyes. When buying fillets, steaks or shellfish, look for firm flesh, clear colour with even colouring and a moist appearance. Fresh fish is best used within a day or two of purchase and can be frozen for 2 to 3 months.

Using: Use a healthy cooking method (baking, roasting, braising, grilling or stir-frying) and allow about 10 minutes of cooking time for every inch of thickness. Like beef, poultry and pork, fish (and shellfish) can be used in an array of ways. You can toss it into a salad, use it in a sandwich, serve it on its own or use it in your favourite recipes.

EGGS

Shopping and Storing: Egg whites (two medium eggs yield about 60ml/2fl oz of egg whites) and egg substitutes are lean-protein, low-

DO I NEED TO BE CONCERNED ABOUT MERCURY IN FISH?

The FSA advises only a small group (women who may become pregnant, pregnant women, nursing mothers and young children) to avoid fish with high levels of contaminants – shark, swordfish or marlin – and to limit any kind of fish to no more than two meals a week. The government also recommends this same group restrict tinned tuna to no more than 4 tins per week (tinned white tuna contains a certain amount of mercury). While this group is *especially* vulnerable to contamination, all of us are at risk and should follow the government's recommendations accordingly.

WHAT IF I'M VEGETARIAN OR VEGAN?

The *Flat Belly Diet* is vegan and vegetarian friendly. We've given you vegan substitutions for the ingredients on the jumpstart plan (page 14). You can also select vegan and vegetarian alternatives, such as beans and lentils, in place of meat and fish in any meal during the 28-day plan. Just be sure to match the calories and keep each meal to about 400 calories. See the list of meat alternatives in the *Flat Belly Diet*-Friendly Products list on page 105.

calorie *Flat Belly Diet* picks. Naturally free of fat and cholesterol, egg whites and egg substitutes have just 25 to 30 calories per 60ml (2fl oz).

Using: Use them in an omelette, a frittata or a quiche; scramble them with veggies, lean meats or low-fat cheese; fill a burrito, a sandwich or a wrap. Egg whites and substitutes can be used in just as many ways as whole eggs.

Dairy

Shopping and Storing: Dairy foods, including milk, yogurt and cheese, are packed with nutrients needed for good health. In fact, research has shown that a diet rich in dairy foods reduces the risk of osteoporosis – a disease that causes bone fractures later in life. But full-fat dairy foods are loaded with calories and artery-clogging saturated fat. What to do? Simply pick low-fat or fat-free dairy products. You'll get all the vitamins and minerals you'd get from whole-milk products but without all of the extra calories and bad-for-you fat. In the supermarket:

- Choose 1% fat milk or skimmed milk.
- Select low-fat or fat-free yogurt with no more than 2 grams of saturated fat per 115g (4oz) serving.
- Choose low-fat or fat-free cheese (including hard cheese, string cheese, cream cheese, cheese spreads and goat's cheese) with no more than 2 or 3 grams of saturated fat per 30g (1oz) serving (115g/4oz of cottage cheese or 60g/2oz of ricotta cheese should have no more than 2 grams of saturated fat).
- Look for low-fat and fat-free versions of other dairy products, including sour cream and crème fraîche.

When shopping for dairy, always compare prices and brands. Many generic brands offer the same quality as the name brands, but for a lot less money. Also check use-by and sell-by dates and buy the product with the latest date.

Using: While yogurt, cheese and milk make a perfect anytime snack all on their own, they can also jazz up just about any MUFA-rich meal. Whip up a smoothie with milk, make a dessert with yogurt and fruit, sprinkle grated cheese over your salad or in your soup or use sliced cheese in a sandwich. The dairy possibilities are endless.

CAN I SUBSTITUTE SOYA FOR DAIRY?

Yes, both soya and dairy products (milk, yogurt, cheese, etc.) provide protein, carbohydrates and nutrients; however, if you pick soya, pick fortified.

Calcium-fortified soya 'dairy' products have nutrient levels similar to cow's-milk products and are the best substitute for real dairy.

IS ORGANIC PRODUCE BEST?

Eating organic produce does help to reduce your exposure to potentially harmful chemicals, and organic farming is better for the environment. However, if money or availability is an issue, limit your organic produce purchases to the 12 fruits and vegetables that are deemed the most contaminated. The 'dirty dozen' are (in order) peaches, apples, peppers, celery, nectarines, strawberries, cherries, lettuce, grapes, pears, spinach and potatoes.

Fruits and Vegetables

Shopping and Storing: Naturally delicious and packed with nutrients and filling fibre, fruits and vegetables are an important part of the *Flat Belly Diet*.

- Choose fresh fruits and vegetables that are firm, unblemished and in season, when they tend to be less expensive.

- Use fresh fruits and veggies within a few days after shopping and use frozen or tinned produce later in the week.

- Choose frozen or tinned fruits and vegetables without added sugar, fat or salt.

- Select whole fruits and vegetables over more expensive pre-cut or prepackaged. When you get home from the supermarket, chop some fresh fruits and vegetables and keep them in the refrigerator so they will be ready to grab for meals and snacks.

- Buy dried fruits and veggies that are processed without added sugar, fat or salt.

- Starchy vegetables like potatoes, beans, lentils, sweetcorn and peas are found not only in the produce aisle but also in the tinned food aisle and the frozen food section. If you choose frozen or tinned starchy vegetables over fresh, be sure to choose no-salt or low-salt varieties and rinse them well before use.

Using: They add crunch, freshness and flavour to any meal or snack. Raw, roasted, steamed, blanched or baked, fruits and vegetables can be tossed into salads, used in sandwiches, served as side dishes, made into salsas and used as desserts. And we're not just talking standard oranges, broccoli or grapes – these days, supermarkets are packed with a wide assortment of exotic fruits and vegetables, and there's no good reason not to grab a few new varieties on every trip to the shops.

Whole Grains

Shopping and Storing: While all grains are good sources of carbohydrates and are naturally low in fat, whole grains – that is, grains that have not had their fibre- and nutrient-rich bran and germ removed by processing – are much, much better. Packed with filling fibre, nutrients and disease-fighting antioxidants and phytochemicals, whole grain products are always a better bet than refined ones.

Look for bread, cereal, couscous, rice, crackers, pasta and other grain products that are 100 per cent whole grain – meaning they contain *no* refined flours. If the label does not say '100 per cent whole grain', flip that pack over and investigate the ingredients list.

○ **Whole grain ingredients to look for:** amaranth, barley, brown rice, buckwheat, bulgur wheat, cracked wheat, millet, oats, popcorn, quinoa, rye, spelt, whole wheat and wild rice

○ **Refined ingredients to avoid:** bleached or unbleached enriched wheat flour, cornmeal, rice flour, semolina or durum flour, white flour and white rice

Don't be fooled by packages that claim to be an 'excellent' or a 'good source of' whole grains or by label terms like *seven-grain, multigrain,*

GOOD CARBS, BAD CARBS

The *Flat Belly Diet* is not a *no*-carb or *low*-carb plan. It's a *balanced* plan. Carbohydrates are your body's main energy source and are necessary in the metabolism of essential nutrients. Any diet that eliminates carbohydrates denies the body what it needs to function properly. However, all carbohydrates are not created equal. Your *Flat Belly Diet* is packed with 'good' (nutrient-dense) carbohydrates like whole grains, fruits, vegetables, low-fat milk and beans, instead of 'bad' (nutrient-poor) carbs such as refined grains and sugary foods like sweets, biscuits, fizzy drinks and cake.

whole grain blend and *made with whole grain*. These foods can contain far more refined grain than whole grain. Always check to see whether the predominant or first ingredient listed is a whole grain.

When deciding on grain products, always compare prices and brands. Like dairy and other packaged products, many generic brands of grains offer the same quality as the name brands, but for a lot less money. Also check use-by and sell-by dates and buy the product with the latest date.

Using: From breakfast (porridge and toast) to lunch (sandwiches, salads and soups) to dinner (pilafs, pastas and side dishes), whole grains can add wholesome flavour to every meal.

THE *FLAT BELLY DIET* STORE CUPBOARD

Now that you have an idea of how to select foods for the *Flat Belly Diet*, here's a summary of a few easy switches to remember the next time you load your shopping trolley. Keep these wholesome ingredients on hand in your cupboard to make it easy for you to prepare a *Flat Belly Diet* meal any time.

BYPASS	BUY INSTEAD
Corn oil or blended vegetable oil	MUFA-rich oils, such as olive or rapeseed oil
Butter or margarine	MUFA-rich spreads such as mashed avocado or hummus
Salted or oil-roasted nuts or seeds	Raw or dry-roasted nuts or seeds without salt
Regular peanut butter	All-natural peanut butter or other nut butter
Milk or white chocolate chips or cocoa powder	Dark chocolate chips
85% lean meat	95% lean meat or vegetarian meat substitutes
Whole or semi-skimmed milk	Skimmed milk or 1% fat milk
Whole-milk cheese or yogurt	Light, low-fat or semi-skimmed cheese or yogurt
Sweetened dried fruit	Unsweetened dried fruit
Tinned fruits or vegetables with added sugar, salt or fat	Tinned or frozen fruits or vegetables with no added sugar, salt or fat
Bleached white flour	Wholemeal or rye flour
Low-fibre cereals and breads	Whole grain cereals and breads with at least 2 to 3 grams of fibre per serving
White, processed pasta	Wholewheat or whole grain pasta
White rice	Brown or wild rice or other whole grains such as barley, millet, oats or rye
Bottled dressings and marinades	MUFA-rich olive oil and vinegar, such as balsamic or rice vinegar
Bottled sauces or spreads	MUFA-rich sauces or spreads such as pesto, tahini or olive tapenade

5.

YOUR ULTIMATE
28-DAY
EATING PLAN

In this chapter, you'll find all of the information you've just learned about MUFA-rich foods and other *Flat Belly Diet* meal building blocks wrapped up into a simple and easy-to-follow plan. This plan takes the guesswork out of creating MUFA-rich meals and makes it super-easy to learn how to eat the *Flat Belly Diet* way. Because this plan was created by a registered dietitian, you can be assured that it supplies all of the nutrients you need. Call it the no-brainer *Flat Belly Diet*.

Your Ultimate 28-Day Eating Plan is, of course, based on the three rules of the *Flat Belly Diet*:

Rule #1: Stick to 400 calories per meal.

Rule #2: Never go more than 4 hours without eating.

Rule #3: Eat a MUFA at every meal.

And it's also based on the guidelines we outlined in Chapter 4: The MUFA Meal Maker Guide:

Guideline #1: Consume no more than 4 grams of saturated fat per meal.

Guideline #2: Ban trans fat.

Guideline #3: Avoid artificial sweeteners, flavourings and preservatives.

Guideline #4: Limit sodium to less than 2,300 milligrams per day.

In this section, you'll find a simple shopping list for each week's worth of meals and a schedule of Quick-and-Easy Meals and Snack Packs, each containing about 400 calories and a MUFA. In each week, you'll see that some of the meals repeat, but trust me, there's enough variety so that you won't get bored. Every week, you'll enjoy three different breakfasts, four lunches, four snacks and five dinners. What's more, you'll get to try six or seven new MUFAs each week. If you do want a different breakfast, lunch, dinner and snack every single day, be my guest. There's no rule against it! However, this 28-day meal plan has been specifically designed to maximize your food budget and prevent wasted leftovers. More variety, of course, means a longer shopping list and more money out of your pocket. So I urge you to give this 28-day plan a try, and if you feel like making a few adjustments, have fun! Chapter 6 contains 30 additional Quick-and-Easy Meals and Snack Packs that can easily be slotted in. Remember, since every meal contains a MUFA and roughly the same number of calories, mixing and matching to create a daily menu you love is easy. And, of course, you can always use recipes from the original *Flat Belly Diet!* book, or create your own based on the guidelines in Chapter 4. One more thing – the 28-day plan has also been designed to save you time; all of the meals can be made in 20 minutes or less and can be made ahead of time. So if you see that Your Ultimate 28-Day Eating Plan calls for Creamy Peanut Soup two times during the week, you can multiply your recipe by two, make one big batch and eat it throughout the week as indicated.

Now tell me, what could be easier than this?

SWAPPING MADE EASY

Feel like having breakfast for dinner? All of the *Flat Belly Diet* meals and snacks are interchangeable, so you can swap or repeat meals to your heart's content. Bear in mind, though, that it's still important to eat a variety of foods to ensure that you get all the nutrients you need. You can also substitute foods you like within a specific meal for those that you don't. If you prefer to have two slices of wholemeal bread instead of a wholewheat tortilla, that's fine! Just match the calories and be sure to choose foods in the same food group to substitute for one another. For example, two slices of bacon are not a substitute for a wholewheat tortilla. But 60g (2oz) fresh mango chunks can substitute for 2 tbsp raisins – they are both fruits and those servings give you about the same number of calories and similar nutritional value.

Here's how to substitute.

1. Swap one meal or snack for another. All of the meals and snacks in the 28-day meal plan and the quick meals and snacks are interchangeable because they have all been designed to stay within the 400-calorie-per-meal range, and they are all nutritionally balanced according to the guidelines in the MUFA Meal Maker Guide.

2. Swap one ingredient for another, but select the same category of food. Substitute a vegetable for a vegetable, a whole grain for a whole

ALL-MUFA MEAL

It's tempting to have an all-MUFA meal or snack. But 400 calories of peanut butter right off the spoon or 400 calories of pecans, and so on, well, that's not how this plan works. First, because MUFAs are high in calories, you won't get enough energy from 400 calories' worth of peanut butter to last you the 4 hours until your next meal. Plus, as much as you might enjoy your MUFA-rich foods, they must be combined with the other foods on your meal plan for you to get enough nutrition from the *Flat Belly Diet*. Plus, pairing your MUFAs with other foods helps slow digestion so you feel fuller longer.

grain, a fruit for a fruit, a MUFA for a MUFA, a dairy for a dairy, a lean protein for a lean protein, or a spice/seasoning for a spice/seasoning. The calories are listed in your meal plan in brackets after the food, so just match the calories and swap the foods. You'll also find three quick reference lists at the back of the book – Your MUFA Serving Chart, Eat These Foods Regularly and Eat These Foods Sparingly – that list serving sizes and calorie counts so that you can easily find a substitute in your category.

MUFA Swaps

If you don't like or can't find a MUFA, don't despair. Swap these like-calorie MUFAs for one another. Look for the MUFA listed in your meal plan and check out the alternatives below to see if a swap makes sense. I've included only a selection of the most common MUFAs with similar calories, so not all MUFAs are listed here. You will find the complete list of MUFAs in Your MUFA Serving Chart on page 116. Go ahead, swap away!

MUFA CALORIES	MUFA SWAPS
About 50	Green olive tapenade, 2 tbsp Green or black olives, 10 large
About 80	Pesto sauce, 1 tbsp Walnuts, 2 tbsp
About 90	Pecans, 2 tbsp Pistachios, 2 tbsp Sunflower seeds, 2 tbsp Black olive tapenade, 2 tbsp
About 100	Cashews, 2 tbsp Avocado, 60g (2oz)
About 110	Almonds, 2 tbsp Brazil nuts, 2 tbsp Hazelnuts, 2 tbsp Pine nuts, 2 tbsp Peanuts, 2 tbsp
About 120	Rapeseed oil, 1 tbsp Flaxseed (linseed) oil (cold-pressed organic), 1 tbsp Olive oil, 1 tbsp Peanut oil, 1 tbsp Safflower oil (high-oleic), 1 tbsp Sesame or soya bean oil, 1 tbsp Sunflower oil (high-oleic), 1 tbsp Walnut oil, 1 tbsp Macadamia nuts, 2 tbsp
About 190	Cashew butter, 2 tbsp Sunflower seed butter, 2 tbsp Peanut butter (natural – crunchy or smooth), 2 tbsp

Meal Building Block Swaps

Swap any of the same category foods in each row for one another. I've listed only the foods that show up in your 28-day plan, but you can feel free to incorporate foods you don't see in your meal plan, such as sweet potatoes, aubergine, kiwi fruit, celery, etc. The list goes on and on! Again, consult the Eat These Foods Regularly and Eat These Foods Sparingly lists at the back of the book for serving sizes and calorie counts to make swapping easy.

BUILDING BLOCK	FOODS
Lean Protein	Tinned wild salmon Cannellini beans Tinned tuna chunks in water Egg whites (or egg substitutes) Hummus Kidney beans Organic roast chicken breast* Organic roast beef* slices Organic turkey breast* slices Vegetarian chicken-style nuggets or goujons Veggie burgers
Dairy	Fat-free cottage cheese Fat-free ricotta cheese Fat-free yogurt** Light string cheese*** Reduced-fat Cheddar cheese Reduced-fat Monterey Jack cheese Reduced-fat grated mozzarella cheese Skimmed milk
Fruits	Apples Bananas Blueberries, fresh or frozen unsweetened Dried cranberries, unsweetened Grapefruit Mangoes Oranges Peaches, fresh or frozen unsweetened Pears Pineapple chunks, tinned in 100% pineapple juice Red or green grapes Strawberries, fresh or frozen unsweetened

BUILDING BLOCK	FOODS
Vegetables	Baby carrots Baby greens Baby spinach Frozen Chinese-style vegetables (includes any combination of bamboo shoots, broccoli, carrots, cauliflower, mushrooms, onions, water chestnuts) Onions Peppers Romaine lettuce Tomatoes
Breads, Cereals and Grains	Brown rice Rolled oats (oatmeal) Whole grain cereal Wholemeal bread Wholemeal crackers Wholemeal English muffins Wholewheat pasta Wholemeal pitta Wholewheat tortillas
Spices, Seasonings and Condiments	Balsamic vinegar Rapeseed oil mayonnaise Dijon mustard Dried herbs and spices Fresh herbs Lemon juice Lime juice

*We call for organic deli meat because it is generally lower in sodium and fat. If you choose to purchase non-organic meat, please look for low-sodium choices.

**Because many fat-free yogurts contain artificial flavourings and sweeteners, please be careful about the brands you choose and read the label carefully!

***We call for light string cheese rather than standard because it is lower in saturated fat and calories. If you have trouble finding light string cheese, though, feel free to substitute with standard string cheese.

SHOPPING MADE EASY

Your Ultimate 28-Day Eating Plan is designed to save you time and money. We've carefully planned the meals so that you will be able to use all of the perishable foods you buy each week (that means no waste), plus we'll help you reuse dry goods and frozen foods throughout the entire plan.

Bear in mind that this means your shopping list in Week 1 is a little longer than it is for the rest of the plan. That's because all of the non-perishable items – condiments, tinned foods, oils, bread products, bars, frozen foods and nuts – that you'll need for all 28 days are included. You may already have a lot of these items to hand, but just in case you don't, you should make a big stock-up trip to a supermarket. Having these essentials handy will make it easier to stay on the *Flat Belly Diet* for the full 28 days.

Keep perishable bread products in the freezer – they'll keep for at least 3 months. Let them defrost on the worktop before using them, or if you're in a hurry, place in the microwave on the defrost setting for about a minute. Store nuts in the freezer or refrigerator (see page 27). When using nuts or seeds in meals, measure them whole, then chop them up for meals.

One final note: Your Ultimate 28-Day Eating Plan was designed for one person, so all of the recipes and shopping lists include just enough food for one. If you're following this plan with your spouse or a house-mate, double the amounts. We always tell you how much of each ingredient you'll be using each week and, in weeks 2, 3 and 4, which ingredients should be left over from the previous week(s) if you were following the plan exactly. (You'll see some frozen and dry goods in Week 1 without an indication of how much you'll be using; those are foods you won't need until later in the plan.)

Note: For dairy or other fresh items that you purchase from week to week, please check the use-by date to be sure they will take you through the whole week.

Note: Fresh herbs are included in some of these recipes. If you need to substitute dried herbs, use one-third of the suggested amount.

Note: Purchasing small amounts of vegetables from the supermarket salad counter may save you time and money.

WEEK 1

DAY	MEAL	RECIPE	MUFA
1	Breakfast	Pumpkin Crunch Cereal	Pumpkin seeds
1	Lunch	Chicken and Apple Salad	Olive oil
1	Snack Pack	Strawberry Chocolate Pancake	Dark chocolate
1	Dinner	Guacamole Dip	Avocado
2	Breakfast	Walnut Apple Pancake	Walnuts
2	Lunch	Chicken Sandwich	Avocado
2	Snack Pack	Apples and Crackers	Almond butter
2	Dinner	Scrambled Egg with Toast	Avocado
3	Breakfast	Mango Strawberry Smoothie	Almond butter
3	Lunch	California Burger	Avocado
3	Snack Pack	Fruit and Nuts	Walnuts
3	Dinner	Dijon Salmon Pitta	Pumpkin seeds
4	Breakfast	**Walnut Apple Pancake**	Walnuts
4	Lunch	Avocado and Salmon Salad	Avocado
4	Snack Pack	**Strawberry Chocolate Pancake**	Dark chocolate
4	Dinner	Waldorf Pitta	Walnuts
5	Breakfast	**Mango Strawberry Smoothie**	Almond butter
5	Lunch	**Chicken and Apple Salad**	Olive oil
5	Snack Pack	**Fruit and Nuts**	Walnuts
5	Dinner	**Guacamole Dip**	Avocado
6	Breakfast	**Pumpkin Crunch Cereal**	Pumpkin seeds
6	Lunch	**California Burger**	Avocado
6	Snack Pack	**Apples and Crackers**	Almond butter
6	Dinner	Chicken Herb Crackers	Walnuts
7	Breakfast	**Mango Strawberry Smoothie**	Almond butter
7	Lunch	**Avocado and Salmon Salad**	Avocado
7	Snack Pack	String Cheese and Fruit Pot	Peanuts
7	Dinner	**Waldorf Pitta**	Walnuts

Bold = Repeated Recipe

WEEK 1

SHOPPING LIST

PRODUCE

- 8 medium apples, any type (using 8)
- 2 medium Granny Smith apples (using 2)
- 5 small bananas (using 5)
- 3 grapefruits (using 3)
- 2 fresh mangoes (using 2)
- 500g (18oz) fresh strawberries or 2 285g (10oz) packs frozen unsweetened strawberries (using 500g/18oz)
- 4 small avocados (using 4)
- 115g (4oz) baby carrots (using 115g/4oz)
- 1 small cucumber (using 1)
- 3 285g (10oz) romaine lettuce packs (using 3 packs)
- 3 medium red peppers (using 3)
- 7 small tomatoes (using 7)
- 1 litre (1³/₄ pints) orange juice, 100% pure
- 1 small bunch fresh coriander (optional) (using 1)
- 1 small bunch fresh parsley (optional) (using 1)
- 1 small bunch fresh tarragon (optional) (using 1)

DAIRY

- 1.2 litres (2 pints) skimmed milk (using 1.2 litres/2 pints)
- 140g (5oz) pack extra light soft cheese wedges (using 5 wedges)
- 170g (6oz) pack light string cheese (using 3 pieces)* (If you are starting this plan immediately after doing the 4-day jumpstart, you should have 2 pieces string cheese left over to use this week.)

EGGS

- 240ml (8fl oz) liquid egg whites (using 120ml/4fl oz)

FROZEN FOODS

- 1 pack wholemeal Scotch pancakes (using 6)
- 285g (10oz) pack frozen unsalted sweetcorn
- 2 285g (10oz) packs frozen shelled edamame (soya beans)
- 2 285g (10oz) packs stir-fry or Chinese-style frozen vegetables (may include broccoli, carrots, cauliflower, mushrooms, water chestnuts; but if this mixture is not available, select a similar mixture),
- 2 340g (12oz) packs vegetarian chicken-style nuggets
- 2 packs veggie burgers (4 in a pack) (using 2)

BREAD/CEREAL

- 400g (14oz) loaf wholemeal bread, 16 slices (using 4 slices)
- 8 wholemeal pitta breads
- 6 wholewheat tortillas
- 230g (8oz) wholewheat pasta, any shape

WEEK 1

- 340g (12oz) box wholemeal crackers, about 1½" square (using 42)
- 500g (18oz) pack rolled oats
- 340g (12oz) box whole grain puffed wheat cereal (using 60g/2oz)

DRY GOODS

- 240ml (8fl oz) bottle rapeseed oil
- 240ml (8fl oz) bottle cold-pressed flaxseed (linseed) oil (If you are starting this plan immediately after doing the 4-day jumpstart, you should have enough flaxseed (linseed) oil to take you through the 28-day plan and don't need to buy any more.)
- 240ml (8fl oz) bottle extra virgin olive oil (using 3 tbsp plus 1 tsp) (If you are starting this plan immediately after doing the 4-day jumpstart, you should have enough olive oil to take you through the 28-day plan and don't need to buy more.)
- 240ml (8fl oz) bottle high-oleic safflower oil
- 180ml (6fl oz) bottle sesame oil
- 240ml (8fl oz) bottle sunflower oil
- 230g (8oz) jar almond butter (using 10 tbsp)
- 230g (8oz) pack roasted or raw unsalted almonds
- 170g (6oz) pack roasted or raw unsalted Brazil nuts

- 60g (2oz) pack raw or roasted unsalted hazelnuts
- 60g (2oz) pack raw unsalted macadamia nuts
- 230g (8oz) pack roasted or raw unsalted pecans
- 170g (6oz) pack roasted or raw unsalted pine nuts
- 115g (4oz) pack raw unsalted pistachios
- 170g (6oz) pack raw unsalted walnut halves (using 14 tbsp)
- 340g (12oz) jar natural peanut butter
- 60g (2oz) pack roasted or raw unsalted peanuts (using 2 tbsp)
- 230g (8oz) pack roasted or raw unsalted pumpkin seeds (using 6 tbsp)
- 2 tbsp (¾oz) sesame seeds
- 90g (3oz) pack raw unsalted sunflower seeds
- 425g (15oz) tin cannellini beans, no salt added
- 425g (15oz) tin kidney beans, no salt added,
- 425g (15oz) jar large green olives
- 425g (15oz) tin plus 200g (7oz) tin large black olives
- 340g (12oz) pack dark chocolate chips (using 90g/3oz)
- 230g (8oz) pack dried unsweetened cranberries

WEEK 1

SHOPPING LIST – CONT.

DRY GOODS (CONT.)

- [ ] 425g (15oz) pack seedless raisins (If you are starting this plan immediately after doing the 4-day jumpstart, you should have enough raisins to take you through the 28-day plan and don't need to buy any more.)

- [ ] 600g (20oz) tin pineapple chunks packed in juice, plus 230g (8oz) tin (using 115g/4oz)

- [ ] 340g (12oz) jar roasted red peppers

- [ ] 230g (8oz) or smaller jar Dijon mustard (using 4 tsp)

- [ ] 230g (8oz) jar rapeseed oil mayonnaise

- [ ] 1 small bottle agave nectar (using 4 tsp)

- [ ] 2 450g (16oz) cartons chicken stock, reduced-sodium

- [ ] 230g (8oz) jar passata, with less than 400 milligrams of sodium per 120ml (4fl oz) serving

MEAL REPLACEMENT BARS

- [ ] Choose 7 meal replacement/ cereal bars. Try to choose bars with organic ingredients and no added sugar. These bars are interchangeable on the plan wherever you see a bar listed with a meal or snack.

MEAT/SEAFOOD

- [ ] 170g (6oz) tin wild salmon or 250g (9oz) fresh salmon (using 170g/6oz) (If you prefer to bake or grill your own salmon for these meals, purchase 90g (3oz) raw salmon for each 60g (2oz) cooked salmon in your meals. The raw weight for fish and meat is a little more than the cooked weight.)

- [ ] 4 90g (3oz) tins tuna chunks in water (or 2 170g/6oz tins or 400g/14oz fresh or frozen tuna steaks – divide into 100g/3½oz portions, store in freezer and defrost and cook as needed)

- [ ] 340g (12oz) pack organic roast chicken breast (using 340g/12oz)**

SPICES AND SEASONINGS

- [ ] 30g (1oz) container ground ginger

- [ ] 30g (1oz) container dried basil

- [ ] 230g (8oz) bottle aged balsamic vinegar (using 4 tbsp)

- [ ] 170g (6oz) bottle rice vinegar (using 2 tbsp)

- [ ] 170g (6oz) bottle sherry vinegar

*We call for light or low-fat string cheese rather than standard because it is lower in saturated fat and calories. If you have trouble finding light or low-fat string cheese, though, feel free to substitute with standard string cheese.

**We call for organic deli meat because it is generally lower in sodium and fat. If you choose to purchase non-organic meat, please look for low-sodium choices.

DAY 1

BREAKFAST

Pumpkin Crunch Cereal: Mix 30g (1oz) puffed wheat cereal (75) with 240ml (8fl oz) skimmed milk (80) and 1 small banana, sliced (90); top with 2 tbsp **pumpkin seeds** (148).

Total calories: 393

LUNCH

Chicken and Apple Salad: Mix 200g (7oz) shredded romaine lettuce (24), 1 small tomato, sliced (12), 1 medium tart apple (such as Granny Smith), diced (95), and 90g (3oz) organic roast chicken breast, sliced into small pieces (75). Toss with 1 tbsp **olive oil** (119) and 2 tbsp balsamic vinegar (10). Crumble 2 small wholemeal crackers over top (36).

Total calories: 371

SNACK PACK

Strawberry Chocolate Pancake: Top 1 wholemeal Scotch pancake (100) with 45g (1½oz) **dark chocolate chips** (207) and place in an oven set to 180°C/350°F/gas 4 for 2 minutes to warm the pancake and slightly melt the chocolate chips. Top with 125g (4½oz) unsweetened strawberries (52).

Total calories: 359

DINNER

Guacamole Dip: Toast 1 wholemeal pitta (140) and cut or break into triangles; dip into a mixture of 60g (2oz) chopped **avocado** (96), 1 tsp agave nectar (20), 1 tsp chopped coriander leaves (0), 2 small tomatoes, chopped (24), and 90g (3oz) finely chopped red pepper (23). Have 1 light string cheese (80).

Total calories: 383

DAY 2

BREAKFAST

Walnut Apple Pancake: Toast 2 wholemeal Scotch pancakes (200) and top with a mixture of 1 medium apple, chopped (95), 1 tsp agave nectar (20) and 2 tbsp **walnuts** (82).

Total calories: 397

LUNCH

Chicken Sandwich: Spread 2 slices wholemeal bread (160) with 60g (2oz) sliced ripe **avocado,** mashed (96); fill with 90g (3oz) organic roast chicken breast (75), 30g (1oz) shredded romaine lettuce (4) and 1 tsp chopped fresh tarragon (0). Have 1 small banana (90).

Total calories: 425

SNACK PACK

Apples and Crackers: Spread 6 small wholemeal crackers (108) with 2 tbsp **almond butter** (200) and serve with 1 medium apple (95).

Total calories: 403

DINNER

Scrambled Egg with Toast: Toast 2 slices wholemeal bread (160) and top with 60g (2oz) sliced **avocado** (96) and 1 small tomato, sliced (12). Scramble 120ml (4fl oz) egg whites (50) with cooking spray, with salt and pepper to taste. Have ½ grapefruit (60).

Total calories: 378

DAY 3

BREAKFAST

Mango Strawberry Smoothie: In a blender, combine 240ml (8fl oz) skimmed milk (80), 2 tbsp **almond butter** (200), 60g (2oz) fresh or frozen unsweetened strawberries (26) and 60g (2oz) unsweetened mango chunks (60).

Total calories: 366

LUNCH

California Burger: Fill 1 wholemeal pitta (140) with 1 cooked veggie burger (100) dressed with 1 tsp Dijon mustard (5); add 30g (1oz) shredded romaine lettuce (4), 90g (3oz) sliced red pepper (23) and 60g (2oz) sliced **avocado** (96).

Total calories: 368

SNACK PACK

Fruit and Nuts: Mix 1 medium apple, diced (95), 1 small banana, sliced (90), and 2 tbsp orange juice (14). Top with 2 tbsp **walnuts** (82). Have 6 small wholemeal crackers (108).

Total calories: 389

DINNER

Dijon Salmon Pitta: Spread 1 wholemeal pitta (140) with 2 tsp Dijon mustard (10) and sprinkle with 2 tbsp **pumpkin seeds** (148), 1 tsp chopped fresh parsley (0) and ¼ cucumber, thinly sliced (9). Fill with 60g (2oz) tinned wild salmon (90).

Total calories: 397

WEEK 1

DAY 4

BREAKFAST

Walnut Apple Pancake: Toast 2 wholemeal Scotch pancakes (200) and top with a mixture of 1 medium apple, chopped (95), 1 tsp agave nectar (20) and 2 tbsp **walnuts** (82).

Total calories: 397

LUNCH

Avocado and Salmon Salad: Mix 200g (7oz) shredded romaine lettuce (24), 60g (2oz) tinned wild salmon (90), 1 grapefruit, sectioned and sliced (120), 60g (2oz) chopped **avocado** (96), 1 tbsp rice vinegar (0) and 2 tsp olive oil (79).

Total calories: 409

SNACK PACK

Strawberry Chocolate Pancake: Top 1 wholemeal Scotch pancake (100) with 45g (1½oz) **dark chocolate chips** (207) and place in an oven set to 180°C/350°F/gas 4 for 2 minutes to warm the pancake and slightly melt the chocolate chips. Top with 125g (4½oz) unsweetened strawberries (52).

Total calories: 359

DINNER

Waldorf Pitta: Split 1 wholemeal pitta (140), spread with 2 extra light soft cheese wedges (70), and fill with 1 medium apple, chopped (95), 2 tbsp **walnuts** (82) and 60g (2oz) shredded romaine lettuce (8).

Total calories: 395

DAY 5

BREAKFAST

Mango Strawberry Smoothie: In a blender, combine 240ml (8fl oz) skimmed milk (80), 2 tbsp **almond butter** (200), 60g (2oz) fresh or frozen unsweetened strawberries (26) and 60g (2oz) unsweetened mango chunks (60).

Total calories: 366

LUNCH

Chicken and Apple Salad: Mix 180g (6oz) shredded romaine lettuce (24), 1 small tomato, sliced (12), 1 medium tart apple (such as Granny Smith), diced (95), and 90g (3oz) organic roast chicken breast, chopped into small pieces (75). Toss with 1 tbsp **olive oil** (119) and 2 tbsp balsamic vinegar (10). Crumble 2 small wholemeal crackers over top (36).

Total calories: 371

SNACK PACK

Fruit and Nuts: Mix 1 medium apple, diced (95), 1 small banana, sliced (90), and 2 tbsp orange juice (14). Top with 2 tbsp **walnuts** (82). Have 6 small wholemeal crackers (108).

Total calories: 389

DINNER

Guacamole Dip: Toast 1 wholemeal pitta (140) and cut into triangles; dip into a mixture of 60g (2oz) chopped **avocado** (96), 1 tsp agave nectar (20), 1 tsp chopped coriander leaves (0), 2 small tomatoes, chopped (24), and 90g (3oz) finely chopped red pepper (23). Have 1 light string cheese (80).

Total calories: 383

DAY 6

BREAKFAST

Pumpkin Crunch Cereal: Mix 30g (1oz) puffed wheat cereal (75) with 240ml (8fl oz) skimmed milk (80) and 1 small banana, sliced (90); top with 2 tbsp **pumpkin seeds** (148).

Total calories: 393

LUNCH

California Burger: Fill 1 wholemeal pitta (140) with 1 cooked veggie burger (100) dressed with 1 tsp Dijon mustard (5); add 30g (1oz) shredded romaine lettuce (4), 90g (3oz) sliced red pepper (23) and 60g (2oz) sliced **avocado** (96).

Total calories: 368

SNACK PACK

Apples and Crackers: Spread 6 small wholemeal crackers (108) with 2 tbsp **almond butter** (200) and serve with 1 medium apple (95).

Total calories: 403

DINNER

Chicken Herb Crackers: Spread 8 small wholemeal crackers (144) with 1 extra light soft cheese wedge (35) and top with 90g (3oz) organic roast chicken breast, cubed (75). Have 60g (2oz) sliced mango (60) topped with 2 tbsp **walnuts** (82).

Total calories: 396

DAY 7

BREAKFAST

Mango Strawberry Smoothie: In a blender, combine 240ml (8fl oz) skimmed milk (80), 2 tbsp **almond butter** (200), 60g (2oz) unsweetened strawberries (26) and 60g (2oz) unsweetened mango chunks (60).

Total calories: 366

LUNCH

Avocado and Salmon Salad: Mix 180g (6oz) shredded romaine lettuce (24), 60g (2oz) tinned wild salmon (90), 1 grapefruit, sectioned and sliced (120), 60g (2oz) chopped **avocado** (96), 1 tbsp rice vinegar (0) and 2 tsp olive oil (79).

Total calories: 409

SNACK PACK

String Cheese and Fruit Pot: Have 1 light string cheese (60), 115g (4oz) pineapple chunks tinned in juice (60), 115g (4oz) baby carrots (50), 6 small wholemeal crackers (108) and 2 tbsp **peanuts** (110).

Total calories: 388

DINNER

Waldorf Pitta: Split 1 wholemeal pitta (140), spread with 2 extra light soft cheese wedges (70) and fill with 1 medium apple, chopped (95), 2 tbsp **walnuts** (82) and 60g (2oz) shredded romaine lettuce (8).

Total calories: 395

WEEK 2

DAY	MEAL	RECIPE	MUFA
8	Breakfast	Vanilla Pecan Parfait	Pecans
8	Lunch	Sesame Chicken Stir-Fry	Sesame oil
8	Snack Pack	Bar and Sunflower Seeds	Sunflower seeds
8	Dinner	Mediterranean Sandwich	Pine nuts
9	Breakfast	Sweet and Savoury Cottage Cheese	Pine nuts
9	Lunch	Edamame Potato Salad	Edamame
9	Snack Pack	Yogurt and Pecans	Pecans
9	Dinner	Tapenade Pasta	Black olive tapenade
10	Breakfast	Cranberry Hazelnut Cereal	Hazelnuts
10	Lunch	Red Pepper Tapenade Wrap	Black olive tapenade
10	Snack Pack	Hummus Dip	Pine nuts
10	Dinner	Baby Green Pitta	Pecans
11	Breakfast	**Vanilla Pecan Parfait**	Pecans
11	Lunch	Chinese Chicken	Sesame oil
11	Snack Pack	Cheese and Crackers	Sunflower seeds
11	Dinner	Tuna Salad	Pine nuts
12	Breakfast	**Sweet and Savoury Cottage Cheese**	Pine nuts
12	Lunch	**Red Pepper Tapenade Wrap**	Black olive tapenade
12	Snack Pack	**Bar and Sunflower Seeds**	Sunflower seeds
12	Dinner	Edamame Stir-Fry	Edamame
13	Breakfast	**Cranberry Hazelnut Cereal**	Hazelnuts
13	Lunch	**Sesame Chicken Stir-Fry**	Sesame oil
13	Snack Pack	**Hummus Dip**	Pine nuts
13	Dinner	**Tapenade Pasta**	Black olive tapenade
14	Breakfast	**Sweet and Savoury Cottage Cheese**	Pine nuts
14	Lunch	**Edamame Potato Salad**	Edamame
14	Snack Pack	**Cheese and Crackers**	Sunflower seeds
14	Dinner	**Baby Green Pitta**	Pecans

Bold = Repeated Recipe

SHOPPING LIST

Note: Beginning this week, you'll notice some items listed in *italics*. If you've been following this plan exactly, you purchased these items in week 1 and should have enough of this food to fulfil what you need this week for the meal plan. We've added this information here just in case you're short on any ingredients for any reason.

PRODUCE

- [ ] 8 medium oranges (using 8)
- [ ] 1.1kg (2½lb) red or green grapes (using 1.1kg/2½lb)
- [ ] 285g (10oz) fresh or frozen unsweetened raspberries (using 285g/10oz)
- [ ] 285g (10oz) pack baby greens (using 1 pack)
- [ ] 2 285g (10oz) packs baby spinach (using 2 packs)
- [ ] 2 medium red peppers (using 2)
- [ ] 2 100g (3½oz) red potatoes (using 2)
- [ ] 1 small bunch spring onions (using 5)
- [ ] 1 lemon (using 1)
- [ ] 1 bunch fresh parsley (optional) (using 1)

DAIRY

- [ ] 1.2 litres (2 pints) skimmed milk (using 1 litre/1¾ pints)
- [ ] 3 170g (6oz) pots fat-free vanilla yogurt
- [ ] 2 450g (16oz) pots fat-free cottage cheese (using 600g/21oz)
- [ ] 230g (8oz) grated reduced-fat mozzarella cheese (using 6 tbsp)
- [ ] *170g (6oz) pack light string cheese**

FROZEN FOODS

- [ ] *Frozen unsalted sweetcorn (using 17g/6oz)*
- [ ] *Frozen shelled edamame (soya beans) (using 685g/1½lb)*
- [ ] *Stir-fry or Chinese-style frozen vegetables (may include broccoli, carrots, cauliflower, mushrooms, water chestnuts; if this mixture is not available, select a similar mixture) (using 685g/1½lb)*
- [ ] *Vegetarian chicken-style nuggets (using 9)*
- [ ] *Veggie burgers (using 2)*

WEEK 2

SHOPPING LIST - CONT.

BREAD/CEREAL

- [ ] Wholemeal bread (using 2 slices)
- [ ] Wholewheat tortillas (using 2)
- [ ] 8 wholemeal pitta breads (using 2)
- [ ] Wholemeal crackers, about 1½" square (using 24)
- [ ] Whole grain puffed wheat cereal (using 150g/5½oz)
- [ ] Wholewheat pasta, any shape (using 300g/10½oz cooked)
- [ ] Brown rice (If you are starting the plan immediately after doing the 4-day jumpstart, you should have enough) (using 60g/2oz cooked)

DRY GOODS

- [ ] Olive oil (using 1 tbsp plus 1 tsp)
- [ ] Raw or roasted unsalted hazelnuts (using 30g/1oz)
- [ ] Sesame oil (using 3 tbsp)
- [ ] Roasted or raw unsalted pecans (using 10 tbsp)
- [ ] Roasted or raw unsalted pine nuts (using 14 tbsp)
- [ ] Raw unsalted sunflower seeds (using 8 tbsp)
- [ ] Sesame seeds (using 2 tbsp)
- [ ] Dried unsweetened cranberries (using 4 tbsp)
- [ ] Jarred roasted red peppers (using 170g/6oz)
- [ ] Rapeseed oil mayonnaise (using 3 tsp)

MEAL REPLACEMENT BARS

- [ ] Meal replacement/cereal bars with organic ingredients and no added sugar (using 2)

MEAT/SEAFOOD

- [ ] Tinned tuna chunks in water (using 170g/6oz) or 340g (12oz) fresh or frozen tuna steaks

SPICES AND SEASONINGS

- *Balsamic vinegar (using 1 tbsp)*
- *Rice vinegar (using 5 tbsp plus 2 tsp)*
- 230g (8oz) container hummus (using 230g/8oz)
- 125g (4½oz) container olive tapenade (You should be able to find this in the refrigerated section near the hummus or deli-style olives) (using 8 tbsp)

*We call for light or low-fat string cheese rather than standard because it is lower in saturated fat and calories. If you have trouble finding light or low-fat string cheese, though, feel free to substitute with standard string cheese.

WEEK 2

DAY 8

BREAKFAST

Vanilla Pecan Parfait: Layer half of these ingredients in this order in a parfait glass; repeat layers, ending with pecans: 30g (1oz) puffed wheat cereal (70), 125g (4½oz) fresh or thawed frozen unsweetened raspberries (70), 170g (6oz) fat-free vanilla yogurt (155) and 2 tbsp **pecans** (90).

Total calories: 385

LUNCH

Sesame Chicken Stir-Fry: Stir-fry 170g (6oz) baby spinach (24) in 1 tbsp toasted **sesame oil** (120), 2 tbsp rice vinegar (0) and 1 tbsp sesame seeds (51) for 2 to 3 minutes. Cook 3 vegetarian chicken-style nuggets (129) in the microwave or according to package directions and add to the mixture; toss to combine and heat for 1 minute. Serve with 1 medium orange (62).

Total calories: 386

SNACK PACK

Bar and Sunflower Seeds: Have 1 meal replacement bar, 2 tbsp **sunflower seeds** (90) and 1 medium orange, sliced (62).

Total calories: 352

DINNER

Mediterranean Sandwich: Mix 75g (3oz) tinned tuna chunks in water, drained (105), with 1 tsp rapeseed oil mayonnaise (33), 1 tbsp rice vinegar (0), 1 tsp chopped fresh parsley (0), 1 tsp lemon juice (1) and 2 tbsp **pine nuts** (113). Fill 2 slices wholemeal bread (160) with the tuna mixture.

Total calories: 412

DAY 9

BREAKFAST

Sweet and Savoury Cottage Cheese: Mix 170g (6oz)
fat-free cottage cheese (180), 2 tbsp toasted **pine nuts**
(113) and 125g (4½oz) red or green grapes, sliced (104).

Total calories: 397

LUNCH

Edamame Potato Salad: Combine 230g (8oz) shelled and
boiled **edamame** (298) with a boiled, then chopped 90g
(3oz) red potato (skin on) (74), 1 tsp rice vinegar (0),
1 tsp rapeseed oil mayonnaise (33) and 2 spring onions,
thinly sliced (10). Season with black pepper.

Total calories: 415

SNACK PACK

Yogurt and Pecans: Have 170g (6oz) fat-free vanilla yogurt
(155) topped with 2 tbsp **pecans** (90). Have 125g (4½oz)
red or green grapes (104).

Total calories: 349

DINNER

Tapenade Pasta: Mix 150g (5½oz) cooked wholewheat
pasta, any shape (131), 2 tbsp **black olive tapenade** (88), 2
tsp olive oil (79), 3 tbsp grated reduced-fat mozzarella
cheese (52) and 45g (1½oz) roasted red peppers (12).
Microwave to warm through and melt the cheese.

Total calories: 362

DAY 10

BREAKFAST

Cranberry Hazelnut Cereal: Mix 45g (1½oz) puffed wheat cereal (105), 240ml (8fl oz) skimmed milk (80), 2 tbsp **hazelnuts** (110) and 2 tbsp dried cranberries (45). Have 1 medium orange (62).

Total calories: 402

LUNCH

Red Pepper Tapenade Wrap: Spread 1 wholewheat tortilla (140) with 2 tbsp **black olive tapenade** (88) and fill with 45g (1½oz) roasted red peppers (12). Have 240ml (8fl oz) skimmed milk (80) and 1 medium orange (62).

Total calories: 382

SNACK PACK

Hummus Dip: Dip 170g (6oz) sliced red peppers (46) into 115g (4oz) hummus (200) sprinkled with 2 tbsp **pine nuts** (113).

Total calories: 359

DINNER

Baby Green Pitta: Fill 1 wholemeal pitta (140) with a mixture of 1 cooked and crumbled veggie burger (100), 75g (2½oz) baby greens (9), 125g (4½oz) cooked sweetcorn (66) and 2 tbsp **pecans** (90).

Total calories: 405

DAY 11

BREAKFAST

Vanilla Pecan Parfait: Layer half of these ingredients in this order in a parfait glass; repeat layers, ending with pecans: 30g (1oz) puffed wheat cereal (70), 125g (4½oz) fresh or thawed frozen unsweetened raspberries (70), 170g (6oz) fat-free vanilla yogurt (155) and 2 tbsp **pecans** (90).

Total calories: 385

LUNCH

Chinese Chicken: Heat 300g (10½oz) frozen Chinese-style vegetables (52) with 1 tbsp **sesame oil** (120); serve with 3 cooked vegetarian chicken-style nuggets (129) and 110g (3½oz) cooked brown rice (109).

Total calories: 410

SNACK PACK

Cheese and Crackers: Have 1 light string cheese (60), 8 small wholemeal crackers (144) and 2 tbsp **sunflower seeds** (90). Have 125g (4½oz) red or green grapes (104).

Total calories: 398

DINNER

Tuna Salad: Mix 125g (4½oz) baby spinach (16), 1 tbsp lemon juice (3), 1 tsp chopped fresh parsley (0) and 1 tbsp balsamic vinegar (10); top with 90g (3oz) tinned tuna chunks in water (105) and 2 tbsp **pine nuts** (113). Have 8 small wholemeal crackers (144).

Total calories: 391

WEEK 2

DAY 12

BREAKFAST

Sweet and Savoury Cottage Cheese: Mix 170g (6oz)
fat-free cottage cheese (180), 2 tbsp toasted **pine nuts**
(113) and 125g (4½oz) red or green grapes, sliced (104).

Total calories: 397

LUNCH

Red Pepper Tapenade Wrap: Spread 1 wholewheat tortilla
(140) with 2 tbsp **black olive tapenade** (88) and fill with
45g (1½oz) roasted red peppers (12). Have 240ml (8fl oz)
skimmed milk (80) and 1 medium orange (62).

Total calories: 382

SNACK PACK

Bar and Sunflower Seeds: Have 1 meal replacement bar,
2 tbsp **sunflower seeds** (90) and 1 medium orange, sliced
(62).

Total calories: 352

DINNER

Edamame Stir-Fry: In a medium frying pan, heat 1 tsp
sesame oil (40), 1 spring onion, sliced (5), 230g (8oz)
shelled and boiled **edamame** (298) and 150g (5½oz)
frozen Chinese-style vegetables (26).

Total calories: 369

DAY 13

BREAKFAST

Cranberry Hazelnut Cereal: Mix 45g (1½oz) puffed wheat cereal (105), 240ml (8fl oz) skimmed milk (80), 2 tbsp **hazelnuts** (110) and 2 tbsp dried cranberries (45). Have 1 medium orange (62).

Total calories: 402

LUNCH

Sesame Chicken Stir-Fry: Stir-fry 90g (3oz) baby spinach (24) in 1 tbsp toasted **sesame oil** (120), 2 tbsp rice vinegar (0) with 1 tbsp sesame seeds (51) for 2 to 3 minutes. Cook 3 vegetarian chicken-style nuggets (129) in the microwave or according to package directions and add to the mixture; toss to combine and heat for 1 minute. Serve with 1 medium orange (62).

Total calories: 386

SNACK PACK

Hummus Dip: Dip 170g (6oz) sliced red peppers (46) into 115g (4oz) hummus (200) sprinkled with 2 tbsp **pine nuts** (113).

Total calories: 359

DINNER

Tapenade Pasta: Mix 150g (5½oz) cooked wholewheat pasta, any shape (131), 2 tbsp **black olive tapenade** (88), 2 tsp olive oil (79), 3 tbsp grated reduced-fat mozzarella cheese (52) and 45g (1½oz) roasted red peppers (12). Microwave to warm through and melt the cheese.

Total calories: 362

WEEK 2

DAY 14

BREAKFAST

Sweet and Savoury Cottage Cheese: Mix 170g (6oz)
fat-free cottage cheese (180), 2 tbsp toasted **pine nuts**
(113) and 125g (4½oz) red or green grapes, sliced (104).

Total calories: 397

LUNCH

Edamame Potato Salad: Combine 230g (8oz) shelled and
boiled **edamame** (298) with a boiled, then chopped 90g
(3oz) red potato (skin on) (74), 1 tsp rice vinegar (0),
1 tsp rapeseed oil mayonnaise (33) and 2 spring onions,
thinly sliced (10). Season with black pepper.

Total calories: 415

SNACK PACK

Cheese and Crackers: Have 1 light string cheese (60), 8
small wholemeal crackers (144) and 2 tbsp **sunflower
seeds** (90). Have 125g (4½oz) red or green grapes (104).

Total calories: 398

DINNER

Baby Green Pitta: Fill 1 wholemeal pitta (140) with a
mixture of 1 cooked and crumbled veggie burger (100),
60g (2oz) baby greens (9), 125g (4½oz) cooked sweetcorn
(66) and 2 tbsp **pecans** (90).

Total calories: 405

WEEK 3

DAY	MEAL	RECIPE	MUFA
15	Breakfast	Bar and Chocolate Chips	Dark chocolate
15	Lunch	Picnic Lunch	Green olives
15	Snack Pack	Crackers and Peanut Butter	Peanut butter
15	Dinner	White Bean Pasta	Pesto
16	Breakfast	Raisin and Nut Cereal	Almonds
16	Lunch	Peanutty Cranberry Wrap	Peanut butter
16	Snack Pack	Deli Snack	Black olive tapenade
16	Dinner	Basil Bean Salad	Olive oil
17	Breakfast	Peach Almond Oatmeal	Almonds
17	Lunch	Creamy Peanut Soup	Peanut butter
17	Snack Pack	Olive and Provolone Sandwich	Green olives
17	Dinner	Veggie Pitta	Sunflower oil
18	Breakfast	**Bar and Chocolate Chips**	Dark chocolate
18	Lunch	**Picnic Lunch**	Green olives
18	Snack Pack	Yogurt and Brazil Nuts	Brazil nuts
18	Dinner	Spinach Sunflower Stir-Fry	Sunflower oil
19	Breakfast	**Raisin and Nut Cereal**	Almonds
19	Lunch	**Cranberry Nut Ricotta Dip**	Brazil nuts
19	Snack Pack	**Olive and Provolone Sandwich**	Green olives
19	Dinner	**White Bean Pasta**	Pesto
20	Breakfast	**Peach Almond Oatmeal**	Almonds
20	Lunch	**Peanutty Cranberry Wrap**	Peanut butter
20	Snack Pack	**Yogurt and Brazil Nuts**	Brazil nuts
20	Dinner	Cheesy Pasta with Spinach	Rapeseed oil
21	Breakfast	**Bar and Chocolate Chips**	Dark chocolate
21	Lunch	**Creamy Peanut Soup**	Peanut butter
21	Snack Pack	**Deli Snack**	Black olive tapenade
21	Dinner	**Veggie Pitta**	Sunflower oil

Bold = Repeated Recipe

WEEK 3

SHOPPING LIST

Note: You'll notice some items listed in *italics*. If you've been following this plan exactly, you purchased these items in week 1 and should have enough of this food to fulfil what we need this week for the meal plan. We've added this information here just in case you're short on any ingredients for any reason.

PRODUCE

- 5 oranges (using 5)
- 285g (10oz) fresh sliced peaches (about 2 medium peaches) or 285g (10oz) pack frozen unsweetened sliced peaches (using 285g/10oz)
- 700g (1½lb) pack baby carrots (using 1 pack)
- 60g (2oz) diced celery (if possible, from the salad bar) or 1 small head celery (using 60g/2oz)
- 285g (10oz) pack baby greens (using 1 pack)
- 285g (10oz) pack baby spinach (using 1 pack)
- 1 lemon (using 1)
- 1 small head garlic (using 1)
- 1 small white or yellow onion (using 1)
- 1 small bunch parsley (optional) (using 1)
- 1 small tomato (using 1)

DAIRY

- 1.2 litres (2 pints) skimmed milk (using 1 litre/1¾ pints)
- 2 170g (6oz) pots fat-free vanilla yogurt
- 140g (5oz) pack extra light soft cheese wedges (using 4 wedges)
- *Grated reduced-fat mozzarella cheese (using 3 tbsp)*
- 60g (2oz) sliced reduced-fat provolone cheese
- 425g (15oz) container fat-free ricotta cheese (using 230g/8oz)
- 230g (8oz) pack light string cheese (using 2 pieces)*

BREAD/CEREAL

- *Wholemeal bread (using 4 slices)*
- *Wholemeal pitta breads (using 3)*
- *Wholewheat tortillas (using 3)*
- *Wholemeal crackers, about 1½" square (using 48)*
- *Rolled oats (using 90g/3oz)*
- *Puffed wheat cereal (using 90g/3oz)*
- *Wholewheat pasta, any shape (using 500g/18oz cooked)*

WEEK 3

DRY GOODS

Rapeseed oil (using 1 tbsp)

Olive oil (using 4 tbsp)

Sunflower oil (using 3 tbsp)

Almonds (using 8 tbsp)

Roasted or raw unsalted Brazil nuts (using 6 tbsp)

Cannellini beans, no salt added (using 200g/7oz)

Peanut butter (using 10 tbsp)

Green olives (using 40)

Dark chocolate chips (using 130g/4½oz)

Dried cranberries (using 8 tbsp)

Raisins (using 11 tbsp)

Jarred roasted red peppers (using 4 tbsp)

Rapeseed oil mayonnaise (using 2 tsp)

Passata (using 115g/4oz)

Reduced-sodium chicken stock (using 450ml/16fl oz)

MEAL REPLACEMENT BARS

Meal replacement/cereal bars with organic ingredients and no added sugar

MEAT/SEAFOOD

Tinned tuna chunks in water (using 170g/6oz)

SPICES AND SEASONINGS

Balsamic vinegar (using 4 tbsp plus 2 tsp)

Sherry vinegar (using 2 tsp)

285g (10oz) container hummus any flavour (using 90g/3oz)

115g (4oz) container pesto (using 2 tbsp)

125g (4½oz) container olive tapenade (You should be able to find this in the refrigerated section near the hummus or deli-style olives) (using 4 tbsp)

*We call for light or low-fat string cheese rather than standard because it is lower in saturated fat and calories. If you have trouble finding light string cheese, though, feel free to substitute with standard string cheese.

WEEK 3

DAY 15

BREAKFAST

Bar and Chocolate Chips: Have 1 meal replacement bar (200) and 45g (1½oz) **dark chocolate chips** (207).

Total calories: 407

LUNCH

Picnic Lunch: Spread 8 small wholemeal crackers (144) with 2 extra light soft cheese wedges (70). Have 10 large **green olives** (50), 60g (2oz) baby carrots (50) and 45g (1½oz) hummus (100).

Total calories: 414

SNACK PACK

Crackers and Peanut Butter: Spread 8 small wholemeal crackers (144) with 2 tbsp crunchy or smooth **peanut butter** (188) and top with 1 tbsp raisins (33).

Total calories: 365

DINNER

White Bean Pasta: Mix 150g (5½oz) cooked wholewheat pasta, any shape (131), with 1 tbsp **pesto sauce** (80), 2 tsp olive oil (79), 115g (4oz) no-salt-added cannellini beans, rinsed and drained (75), and 2 tbsp roasted red peppers (6). Microwave to warm through.

Total calories: 377

DAY 16

BREAKFAST

Raisin and Nut Cereal: Mix 45g (1½oz) puffed wheat cereal (105), 240ml (8fl oz) skimmed milk (80), 2 tbsp **almonds** (109) and 2 tbsp raisins (66).

Total calories: 360

LUNCH

Peanutty Cranberry Wrap: Spread 1 wholewheat tortilla (140) with 2 tbsp crunchy or smooth **peanut butter** (188) and 2 tbsp dried cranberries (35). Have 60g (2oz) carrots (50).

Total calories: 413

SNACK PACK

Deli Snack: Spread 8 small wholemeal crackers (144) with 2 tbsp **black olive tapenade** (88). Serve with 60g (2oz) baby carrots (50) and 90g (3oz) tinned tuna chunks in water (105) mixed with 1 tsp rapeseed oil mayonnaise (33).

Total calories: 420

DINNER

Basil Bean Salad: Mix 140g (5oz) rinsed and drained cannellini beans (225), 1 small tomato, chopped (12), 1 tbsp **olive oil** (119), 2 tbsp balsamic vinegar (10) and ¼ tsp dried basil (0).

Total calories: 366

WEEK 3

DAY 17

BREAKFAST

Peach Almond Oatmeal: Cook 45g (1½oz) rolled oats with water to the consistency of your choice (150) and top with 2 tbsp **almonds** (109) and 115g (4oz) fresh or thawed frozen unsweetened sliced peaches (60). Have 240ml (8fl oz) skimmed milk (80).

Total calories: 399

LUNCH

Creamy Peanut Soup: Sauté 30g (1oz) chopped celery (4) and 2 tbsp chopped onion (9) in 1 tsp olive oil (39) for 3 to 5 minutes or until soft. Add 240ml (8fl oz) reduced-sodium chicken stock (17), 1 tsp sherry vinegar (0) and 1 tsp lemon juice (1). Bring to the boil, then reduce heat and simmer for 5 to 7 minutes. Just before serving, stir in 2 tbsp **peanut butter** (188). Mix 60g (2oz) fat-free ricotta cheese (50) and 1 tbsp raisins (33); use as a dip for ½ wholemeal pitta (70), toasted and cut into triangles.

Total calories: 410

SNACK PACK

Olive and Provolone Sandwich: Mix 10 **green olives,** sliced (50), with 1 chopped garlic clove (5), 1 tsp balsamic vinegar (3), 1 tsp olive oil (39) and 1 tsp chopped fresh parsley (0). Let marinate overnight; fill 2 slices wholemeal bread (160) with the mixture and add 30g (1oz) reduced-fat provolone cheese (81). Serve with 1 medium orange, sliced (62).

Total calories: 400

DINNER

Veggie Pitta: Fill 1 wholemeal pitta (140) with a mixture of 15g (½oz) baby spinach (4), 75g (2½oz) baby greens (9), 30g (1oz) baby carrots, chopped (25), 1 tbsp **sunflower oil** (120), 1 tbsp balsamic vinegar (10) and 1 light string cheese, chopped (60).

Total calories: 368

DAY 18

BREAKFAST

Bar and Chocolate Chips: Have 1 meal replacement bar (200) and 45g (1½oz) **dark chocolate chips** (207).

Total calories: 407

LUNCH

Picnic Lunch: Spread 8 small wholemeal crackers (144) with 2 extra light soft cheese wedges (70). Have 10 large **green olives** (50), 60g (2oz) baby carrots (50) and 60g (2oz) hummus (100).

Total calories: 414

SNACK PACK

Yogurt and Brazil Nuts: Top 170g (6oz) fat-free vanilla yogurt (155) with 2 tbsp **Brazil nuts** (110) and 2 tbsp raisins (66). Have 1 medium orange (62).

Total calories: 393

DINNER

Spinach Sunflower Stir-Fry: Heat 90g (3oz) baby spinach (24) in 1 tbsp **sunflower oil** (120); add 1 medium orange, sectioned (62) and 2 tbsp dried cranberries (45). Have 8 small wholemeal crackers (144).

Total calories: 395

WEEK 3

DAY 19

BREAKFAST

Raisin and Nut Cereal: Mix 45g (1½oz) puffed wheat cereal (105), 240ml (8fl oz) skimmed milk (80), 2 tbsp **almonds** (109) and 2 tbsp raisins (66).

Total calories: 360

LUNCH

Cranberry Nut Ricotta Dip: Toast 1 wholewheat tortilla (140) in a 180°C/350°F/gas 4 oven for 2 minutes, until crisp; break into pieces. Mix 115g (4oz) fat-free ricotta cheese (100), 2 tbsp dried cranberries (35) and 2 tbsp **Brazil nuts,** chopped (110). Dip toasted pieces of tortilla into ricotta mixture.

Total calories: 385

SNACK PACK

Olive and Provolone Sandwich: Mix 10 **green olives**, sliced (50), with 1 chopped garlic clove (5), 1 tsp balsamic vinegar (3), 1 tsp olive oil (33) and 1 tsp chopped fresh parsley (0). Let marinate overnight; fill 2 slices wholemeal bread (160) with the mixture and add 30g (1oz) reduced-fat provolone cheese (81). Serve with 1 medium orange, sliced (62).

Total calories: 394

DINNER

White Bean Pasta: Mix 150g (5½oz) cooked wholewheat pasta, any shape (131), with 1 tbsp **pesto sauce** (80), 2 tsp olive oil (79), 115g (4oz) no-salt-added cannellini beans, rinsed and drained (75), and 2 tbsp roasted red peppers (6). Microwave to warm through.

Total calories: 377

DAY 20

BREAKFAST

Peach Almond Oatmeal: Cook 45g (1½oz) rolled oats with water to the consistency of your choice (150) and top with 2 tbsp **almonds** (109) and 115g (4oz) fresh or thawed frozen unsweetened sliced peaches (60). Have 240ml (8fl oz) skimmed milk (80).

Total calories: 399

LUNCH

Peanutty Cranberry Wrap: Spread 1 wholewheat tortilla (140) with 2 tbsp crunchy or smooth **peanut butter** (188) and 2 tbsp dried cranberries (35). Have 60g (2oz) baby carrots (50).

Total calories: 413

SNACK PACK

Yogurt and Brazil Nuts: Top 170g (6oz) fat-free vanilla yogurt (155) with 2 tbsp **Brazil nuts** (110) and 2 tbsp raisins (66). Have 1 medium orange (62).

Total calories: 393

DINNER

Cheesy Pasta with Spinach: Mix 150g (5½oz) cooked wholewheat pasta, any shape (131), 1 tbsp **rapeseed oil** (124), 3 tbsp grated reduced-fat mozzarella cheese (52), 115g (4oz) baby spinach (8) and 30g (1oz) passata (60). Serve hot.

Total calories: 375

WEEK 3

DAY 21

BREAKFAST

Bar and Chocolate Chips: Have 1 meal replacement bar (200) and 45g (1½oz) **dark chocolate chips** (207).

Total calories: 407

LUNCH

Creamy Peanut Soup: Sauté 30g (1oz) chopped celery (4) and 2 tbsp chopped onion (9) in 1 tsp olive oil (39) for 3 to 5 minutes or until soft. Add 240ml (8fl oz) reduced-sodium chicken stock (17), 1 tsp sherry vinegar (0) and 1 tsp lemon juice (1). Bring to the boil, then reduce heat and simmer for 5 to 7 minutes. Just before serving, stir in 2 tbsp **peanut butter** (188). Mix 60g (2oz) fat-free ricotta cheese (50) and 1 tbsp raisins (33); use as a dip for ½ wholemeal pitta (70), toasted and cut into triangles.

Total calories: 410

SNACK

Deli Snack: Spread 8 small wholemeal crackers (144) with 2 tbsp **black olive tapenade** (88). Serve with 60g (2oz) baby carrots (50) and 90g (3oz) tinned tuna chunks in water (105) mixed with 1 tsp rapeseed oil mayonnaise (33).

Total calories: 420

DINNER

Veggie Pitta: Fill 1 wholemeal pitta (140) with a mixture of 15g (½oz) baby spinach (4), 75g (2½oz) baby greens (9), 30g (1oz) baby carrots, chopped (25), 1 tbsp **sunflower oil** (120), 1 tbsp balsamic vinegar (10) and 1 light string cheese, chopped (60).

Total calories: 368

WEEK 4

DAY	MEAL	RECIPE	MUFA
22	Breakfast	Chocolate Raspberry Yogurt	Dark chocolate
22	Lunch	Roast Beef Pitta	Black olives
22	Snack Pack	Cottage Cheese and Pineapple	Pecans
22	Dinner	Dijon Garden Burger Roll-Up	Pistachios
23	Breakfast	Bar and Hazelnuts	Hazelnuts
23	Lunch	Safflower Chicken Stir-Fry	Safflower oil
23	Snack Pack	Strawberry Chocolate Oatmeal	Dark chocolate
23	Dinner	Hearty Salad	Flaxseed (linseed) oil
24	Breakfast	Pistachio Cereal	Pistachios
24	Lunch	Macadamia Pear Salad	Macadamia nuts
24	Snack Pack	Ginger Tahini Dip with Vegetables	Tahini
24	Dinner	Deli Wrap	Black olives
25	Breakfast	**Chocolate Raspberry Yogurt**	Dark chocolate
25	Lunch	Refried Bean Wrap	Flaxseed (linseed) oil
25	Snack Pack	**Cottage Cheese and Pineapple**	Pecans
25	Dinner	Pistachio Herb Wrap	Pistachios
26	Breakfast	**Bar and Hazelnuts**	Hazelnuts
26	Lunch	**Roast Beef Pitta**	Black olives
26	Snack Pack	**Ginger Tahini Dip with Vegetables**	Tahini
26	Dinner	**Hearty Salad**	Flaxseed (linseed) oil
27	Breakfast	**Pistachio Cereal**	Pistachios
27	Lunch	**Safflower Chicken Stir-Fry**	Safflower oil
27	Snack Pack	**Strawberry Chocolate Oatmeal**	Dark chocolate
27	Dinner	**Deli Wrap**	Black olives
28	Breakfast	**Chocolate Raspberry Yogurt**	Dark chocolate
28	Lunch	**Macadamia Pear Salad**	Macadamia nuts
28	Snack Pack	**Cottage Cheese and Pineapple**	Pecans
28	Dinner	Roast Beef Wrap	Tahini

Bold = Repeated Recipe

WEEK 4

SHOPPING LIST

Note: You'll notice some items listed in *italics*. If you've been following this plan exactly, you purchased these items in week 1 and should have enough of this food to fulfil what you need this week for the meal plan. We've added this information here just in case you're short on any ingredients for any reason.

PRODUCE

- 6 medium pears (using 6)
- 425g (15oz) fresh strawberries or 2 285g (10oz) packs frozen unsweetened strawberries (using 425g/15oz)
- 425g (15oz) fresh raspberries or 2 285g (10oz) packs frozen unsweetened raspberries (using 425g/15oz)
- 340g (12oz) pack baby carrots (using 1 pack)
- 285g (10oz) pack baby greens (using 1 pack)
- 2 275g (9oz) packs baby spinach (using 2 packs)
- 1 medium orange pepper (using 1)
- 5 small tomatoes (using 5)
- 1 medium onion (using 1)
- 1 bunch coriander (optional) (using 1)

DAIRY

- 1.2 litres (2 pints) skimmed milk (using 1.2 litres/2 pints)
- 3 170g (6oz) pots fat-free Greek yogurt (using 3 pots)
- 170g (6oz) pack extra light soft cheese wedges (using 6 wedges)
- 700g (1½lb) fat-free cottage cheese (using 360g/12oz)
- *Light string cheese (using 2 pieces)**

FROZEN FOODS

- *Vegetarian chicken-style nuggets (using 8)*
- *Veggie burgers (using 1)*

BREAD/CEREAL

- *Wholemeal pitta breads (using 4)*
- 6 wholewheat tortillas (using 4)
- *Rolled oats (using 90g/3oz)*
- *Whole grain puffed wheat cereal (using 90g/3oz)*

WEEK 4

DRY GOODS

- Flaxseed (linseed) oil, cold-pressed (using 3 tbsp)
- Safflower oil (using 2 tbsp)
- Sesame oil (using 6 tsp)
- Hazelnuts (using 4 tbsp)
- Raw unsalted macadamia nuts (using 4 tbsp)
- Roasted or raw unsalted pecans (using 6 tbsp)
- Raw unsalted pistachios (using 8 tbsp)
- Kidney beans (using 60g/2oz)
- Large black olives (using 50)
- Dark chocolate chips (using 230g/8oz)
- Pineapple chunks tinned in juice (using 700g/1½lb)
- Raisins (using 8 tbsp)
- Dijon mustard (using 2 tsp)
- Rapeseed oil mayonnaise (using 5 tsp)
- Agave nectar (using 5 tsp)

MEAL REPLACEMENT BARS

- Meal replacement/cereal bars with organic ingredients and no added sugar (using 7)

MEAT/SEAFOOD

- 2 170g (6oz) packs organic roast beef slices (using 320g/11oz)**
- 230g (8oz) pack organic turkey breast slices (using 230g/8oz)**

SPICES AND SEASONINGS

- Balsamic vinegar (using 2 tbsp)
- Rice vinegar (using 3 tbsp plus 1 tsp)
- Ground ginger (using ½ tsp)
- 230g (8oz) container hummus (using 115g/4oz)
- 115g (4oz) container tahini (using 6 tbsp)

*We call for light or low-fat string cheese rather than standard because it is lower in saturated fat and calories. If you have trouble finding light string cheese, though, feel free to substitute with standard string cheese.

**We call for organic deli meat because it is generally lower in sodium and fat. If you choose to purchase non-organic meat, please look for low-sodium choices.

WEEK 4

DAY 22

BREAKFAST

Chocolate Raspberry Yogurt: Mix 170g (6oz) fat-free Greek yogurt (80) with 45g (1½oz) **dark chocolate chips** (207) and 115g (4oz) fresh or thawed frozen unsweetened raspberries (70). Drizzle with 1 tsp agave nectar (20).

Total calories: 377

LUNCH

Roast Beef Pitta: Spread 1 wholemeal pitta (140) with 2 tsp rapeseed oil mayonnaise (66) and fill with 10 sliced **black olives** (50) and 115g (4oz) organic roast beef slices (129).

Total calories: 385

SNACK PACK

Cottage Cheese and Pineapple: Mix 170g (6oz) fat-free cottage cheese (180), 230g (8oz) pineapple chunks tinned in juice, drained (120), and 2 tbsp **pecans** (90).

Total calories: 390

DINNER

Dijon Garden Burger Roll-Up: Fill 1 wholewheat tortilla (140) with 1 cooked and crumbled veggie burger (100) dressed with 2 tsp Dijon mustard (10) and 1 tsp rapeseed oil mayonnaise (33), 15g (½oz) baby spinach (4), 1 small tomato, diced (12) and 2 tbsp **pistachios** (88).

Total calories: 387

DAY 23

BREAKFAST

Bar and Hazelnuts: Have 1 meal replacement bar (180) with 2 tbsp **hazelnuts** (110), 1 tbsp raisins (33) and 240ml (8fl oz) skimmed milk (80).

Total calories: 403

LUNCH

Safflower Chicken Stir-Fry: Sauté 30g (1oz) diced onion (16) and 30g (1oz) chopped baby carrots (25) in 1 tbsp **high-oleic safflower oil** (120) until onions are translucent, about 4 to 5 minutes. Heat 4 vegetarian chicken-style nuggets (172) according to the package directions; add to the pan with 90g (3oz) baby spinach (24) and stir until spinach is wilted, about 1 minute.

Total calories: 357

SNACK PACK

Strawberry Chocolate Oatmeal: Cook 45g (1½oz) rolled oats with water to the consistency of your choice (150); stir in 115g (4oz) fresh or thawed frozen unsweetened strawberries (52) and 45g (1½oz) **dark chocolate chips** (207).

Total calories: 409

DINNER

Hearty Salad: Mix 140g (5oz) baby greens (27), 1 small tomato, diced (12), 30g (1oz) baby carrots, chopped (25), 1 light string cheese, chopped (60) and 5 large black olives, chopped (25). Drizzle with 1 tbsp cold-pressed organic **flaxseed (linseed) oil** (120) and 1 tbsp balsamic vinegar (5). Serve with a toasted wholemeal pitta (140).

Total calories: 414

DAY 24

BREAKFAST

Pistachio Cereal: Mix 60g (2oz) puffed wheat cereal (140), 240ml (8fl oz) skimmed milk (80), 2 tbsp **pistachios** (88) and 2 tbsp raisins (66).

Total calories: 374

LUNCH

Macadamia Pear Salad: Mix 90g (3oz) baby spinach (24), 1 medium pear, sliced (103), 1 tbsp raisins (33), 1 small tomato, diced (12), 2 tsp sesame oil (80), 1 tbsp rice vinegar (0) and 2 tbsp **macadamia nuts** (120).

Total calories: 372

SNACK PACK

Ginger Tahini Dip with Vegetables: Combine 2 tbsp **tahini** (178) with 1 tsp chopped fresh coriander (0), 1 tsp toasted sesame oil (33), 1 tsp agave nectar (20) and ¼ tsp ground ginger (0) as dip for 90g (3oz) sliced orange peppers (23). Have with 1 medium pear (103), sliced and spread with 2 extra light soft cheese wedges (70).

Total calories: 426

DINNER

Deli Wrap: Spread 115g (4oz) organic turkey breast slices (131) with 60g (2oz) hummus (100), sprinkle with 10 sliced **black olives** (50) and roll up. Have 1 medium pear (103).

Total calories: 384

DAY 25

BREAKFAST

Chocolate Raspberry Yogurt: Mix 170g (6oz) fat-free Greek yogurt (80) with 45g (1½oz) **dark chocolate chips** (207) and 115g (4oz) fresh or thawed frozen unsweetened raspberries (70). Drizzle with 1 tsp agave nectar (20).

Total calories: 377

LUNCH

Refried Bean Wrap: Warm 30g (1oz) diced onion (16), 1 tbsp balsamic vinegar (5) and 1 tbsp cold-pressed organic **flaxseed (linseed) oil** (120) in a frying pan. Stir in 60g (2oz) mashed no-salt-added kidney beans (100). Spread on 1 wholewheat tortilla (140).

Total calories: 381

SNACK PACK

Cottage Cheese and Pineapple: Mix 170g (6oz) fat-free cottage cheese (180), 230g (8oz) pineapple chunks tinned in juice, drained (120) and 2 tbsp **pecans** (90).

Total calories: 390

DINNER

Pistachio Herb Wrap: Spread 1 wholewheat tortilla (140) with 2 extra light soft cheese wedges (70) and sprinkle with 2 tbsp **pistachios** (88). Have 240ml (8fl oz) skimmed milk (80).

Total calories: 378

WEEK 4

DAY 26

BREAKFAST

Bar and Hazelnuts: Have 1 meal replacement bar (180) with 2 tbsp **hazelnuts** (110), 1 tbsp raisins (33) and 240ml (8fl oz) skimmed milk (80).

Total calories: 403

LUNCH

Roast Beef Pitta: Spread 1 wholemeal pitta (140) with 2 tsp rapeseed oil mayonnaise (66) and fill with 10 sliced **black olives** (50) and 115g (4oz) organic roast beef slices (129).

Total calories: 385

SNACK PACK

Ginger Tahini Dip with Vegetables: Combine 2 tbsp **tahini** (178) with 1 tsp chopped fresh coriander (0), 1 tsp toasted sesame oil (33), 1 tsp agave nectar (20) and ¼ tsp ground ginger (0) as a dip for 90g (3oz) sliced orange peppers (23). Have 1 medium pear (103), sliced and spread with 2 extra light soft cheese wedges (70).

Total calories: 426

DINNER

Hearty Salad: Mix 170g (6oz) baby greens (27), 1 small tomato, diced (12), 30g (1oz) baby carrots, chopped (25), 1 light string cheese, chopped (60) and 5 large black olives, chopped (25). Drizzle with 1 tbsp cold-pressed organic **flaxseed (linseed) oil** (120) and 1 tbsp balsamic vinegar (5). Serve with a toasted wholemeal pitta (140).

Total calories: 414

DAY 27

BREAKFAST

Pistachio Cereal: Mix 60g (2oz) puffed wheat cereal (140), 240ml (8fl oz) skimmed milk (80), 2 tbsp **pistachios** (88) and 2 tbsp raisins (66).

Total calories: 374

LUNCH

Safflower Chicken Stir-Fry: Sauté 30g (1oz) diced onion (16) and 30g (1oz) chopped baby carrots (25) in 1 tbsp **high-oleic safflower oil** (120) until onions are translucent, about 4 to 5 minutes. Heat 4 vegetarian chicken-style nuggets (172) according to the package directions; add to the pan with 90g (3oz) baby spinach (24) and stir until spinach is wilted, about 1 minute.

Total calories: 357

SNACK PACK

Strawberry Chocolate Oatmeal: Cook 45g (1½oz) rolled oats with water to the consistency of your choice (150); stir in 115g (4oz) fresh or thawed frozen unsweetened strawberries (52) and 45g (1½oz) **dark chocolate chips** (207).

Total calories: 409

DINNER

Deli Wrap: Spread 115g (4oz) organic turkey breast slices (131) with 60g (2oz) hummus (100), sprinkle with 10 sliced **black olives** (50) and roll up. Have 1 medium pear (103).

Total calories: 384

WEEK 4

DAY 28

BREAKFAST

Chocolate Raspberry Yogurt: Mix 170g (6oz) fat-free Greek yogurt (80) with 45g (1½oz) **dark chocolate chips** (207) and 115g (4oz) fresh or thawed frozen unsweetened raspberries (70). Drizzle with 1 tsp agave nectar (20).

Total calories: 377

LUNCH

Macadamia Pear Salad: Mix 90g (3oz) baby spinach (24), 1 medium pear, sliced (103), 1 tbsp raisins (33), 1 small tomato, diced (12), 2 tsp sesame oil (80), 1 tbsp rice vinegar (0) and 2 tbsp **macadamia nuts** (120).

Total calories: 372

SNACK PACK

Cottage Cheese and Pineapple: Mix 170g (6oz) fat-free cottage cheese (180), 230g (8oz) pineapple chunks tinned in juice, drained (120), and 2 tbsp **pecans** (90).

Total calories: 390

DINNER

Roast Beef Wrap: Spread 1 wholewheat tortilla (140) with 2 tbsp **tahini** (178); fill with 90g (3oz) organic roast beef slices (97) and 15g (½oz) baby spinach (4).

Total calories: 419

6.

ADDITIONAL
QUICK-AND-EASY
MEALS &
SNACK PACKS

When you need some variation from Your Ultimate 28-Day Eating Plan, look no further than these Quick-and-Easy Meals and Snack Packs. You can substitute any of these for any meal on the diet. They're all simple, throw-together options with minimal ingredients, yet they're tasty and healthy. What a great combination!

BREAKFASTS

Tomato Basil Ricotta Wrap:
Fill 1 wholewheat tortilla (140)
with a mixture of 1 small
tomato, chopped (12),
1 tsp chopped fresh or
1/3 tsp dried basil (0), 115g
(4oz) fat-free ricotta cheese
(100) and 1 tbsp **olive oil**
(119).

■ Total calories: 371

Raisin Almond Wrap: Spread
1 wholewheat tortilla (140)
with 2 tbsp **almond butter**
(200) and sprinkle with 2 tbsp
raisins (66).

■ Total calories: 406

**Peanut Butter Toast and
Strawberries:** Spread 2 slices
toasted wholemeal bread (160)
with 2 tbsp crunchy or smooth
peanut butter (188). Serve with
115g (4oz) sliced fresh or
thawed frozen unsweetened
strawberries (52).

■ Total calories: 400

Pumpkin Raisin Wrap: Mix
90g (3oz) fat-free cottage
cheese (90) with 1/4 tsp ground
cinnamon (0), 1 tbsp raisins
(33) and 2 tbsp **pumpkin
seeds** (148). Fill 1 wholewheat
tortilla (140) with the mixture.

■ Total calories: 411

Apple Cobbler: Mix 45g
(1 1/2oz) puffed wheat cereal
(105) with 1 medium apple,
chopped (95), 2 tbsp **walnuts**
(82) and 240ml (8fl oz)
skimmed milk (80). Heat in the
microwave on high for 1 minute
or until warm. Sprinkle with
1/4 tsp each of ground
cinnamon (0) and ground
nutmeg (0).

■ Total calories: 362

LUNCHES

Cheesy Roast Beef Muffin:
Spread 1 toasted wholemeal
English muffin (140) with 1
extra light soft cheese wedge
(35) and 2 tbsp **cashews** (148).
Fill with 60g (2oz) organic
roast beef slices (65).

■ Total calories: 388

Spiced Edamame: Mix 230g
(8oz) shelled and boiled
edamame (298) with 1/4 tsp
ground cumin (0) and 1 shake
of cayenne pepper (0). Serve
with 110g (3 1/2oz) cooked
brown rice (109).

■ Total calories: 407

Grapefruit Walnut Salad: Mix 170g (6oz) shredded romaine lettuce (24), 2 tbsp **walnuts** (82), 1 grapefruit, sectioned (120), and ½ tsp ground black pepper (0). Serve with 2 slices toasted wholemeal bread (160) spread with 2 tbsp mashed avocado (48).

■ Total calories: 434

Walnut Raisin Pitta: Fill 1 wholemeal pitta (140) with a mixture of 2 tbsp **walnuts** (82), 1 tbsp raisins (33), 90g (3oz) organic chicken breast slices (75), 1 small tomato, diced (12), 30g (1oz) shredded romaine lettuce (4) and 1 tsp olive oil (39).

■ Total calories: 385

Monterey Corn Tortilla: Sprinkle 3 small corn tortillas (171) with 4 tbsp grated Monterey Jack cheese (81); heat under the grill or in the oven to warm. Top with 60g (2oz) salsa (18), 60g (2oz) sliced **avocado** (96) and 30g (1oz) baby spinach (8).

■ Total calories: 374

DINNERS

Mexican Pitta: Fill 1 wholemeal pitta (140) with a mixture of 60g (2oz) rinsed and drained kidney beans (75), 2 tbsp salsa (9), 1 tbsp **olive oil** (119), 30g (1oz) shredded romaine lettuce (4) and 2 tbsp grated reduced-fat Cheddar cheese (40).

■ Total calories: 387

Peanut Mango Chutney Roll: Spread 1 wholewheat tortilla (140) with 1 tsp peanut butter (31). Top with 2 tbsp **peanuts** (110), 60g (2oz) organic chicken breast slices (50) and 115g (4oz) mango chunks (60) sprinkled with 1 tsp lime juice (1).

■ Total calories: 392

Speedy Chicken Satay: Fill 1 wholewheat tortilla (140) with a mixture of 115g (4oz) organic chicken breast slices (100), 2 tbsp **peanuts** (110), 1 tsp chopped fresh tarragon (0) and 2 tbsp fat-free plain yogurt (15).

■ Total calories: 365

Pecan Coriander Turkey:
Sauté 115g (4oz) raw minced turkey breast (120) in 2 tsp olive oil (78) until cooked. Stir in 50g (1¾oz) cooked brown rice (55), 2 tbsp **pecans** (90), 1 tsp chopped coriander (0), ½ tsp chipotle chilli pepper (0) and ¼ tsp ground black pepper (0). Heat through. Have 90g (3oz) red or green grapes (52).

■ Total calories: 395

Cranberry Pistachio Pitta: Fill 1 wholemeal pitta (140) with a mixture of 115g (4oz) fat-free ricotta cheese (90), 1 tsp agave nectar (20), 2 tbsp dried cranberries (45) and 2 tbsp **pistachios** (88).

■ Total calories: 383

Salmon and Brown Rice: Mix 115g (4oz) tinned wild salmon (180), 2 tsp olive oil (78), 2 tbsp **walnuts** (82) and 75g (2½oz) cooked brown rice (73).

■ Total calories: 413

Turkey Roll-Up: Spread 1 wholewheat tortilla (140) with 1 tbsp rapeseed oil mayonnaise (99) and fill with 90g (3oz) organic turkey breast slices (75), 2 tbsp **walnuts** (82), 1 tsp raisins (11) and 30g (1oz) shredded romaine lettuce (4).

■ Total calories: 411

Bean and Rice Salad: Top 110g (3½oz) cooked brown rice (109) with a mixture of 90g (3oz) rinsed and drained pinto beans (83), 60g (2oz) chopped **avocado** (96), 1 small tomato, diced (12), 2 tsp olive oil (78), 2 tbsp salsa (9), 2 tbsp lime juice (6) and a shake of black pepper (0).

■ Total calories: 393

California Pitta: Fill 1 wholemeal pitta (140) with 115g (4oz) organic roast turkey slices (100), 1 small tomato, diced (12), 60g (2oz) chopped **avocado** (96) and 15g (½ oz) baby spinach (4).

■ Total calories: 352

Chicken, Cheese and Olive Wrap: Fill 1 wholewheat tortilla (140) with 4 tbsp grated reduced-fat Monterey Jack cheese (81), 10 large **black olives,** sliced (50), and 115g (4oz) organic chicken breast slices (100).

■ Total calories: 371

SNACK PACKS

Pancake with Almond Butter Spread: Top 1 toasted wholemeal Scotch pancake (100) with 2 tbsp **almond butter** (200) blended with 2 tbsp fat-free plain yogurt (15). Top with 115g (4oz) sliced fresh or thawed frozen unsweetened strawberries (52).

■ Total calories: 367

Edamame Salad: Mix together 230g (8oz) shelled and boiled **edamame** (298), 1 tbsp lemon juice (4), 1 tsp olive oil (33), 125g (4¹/₂oz) cooked sweetcorn (66) and 45g (1¹/₂oz) chopped red pepper (12).

■ Total calories: 413

Bar and Pecans: Have 1 meal replacement bar (180) with 2 tbsp **pecans** (90), 115g (4oz) pineapple chunks tinned in juice (60) and 4 small wholemeal crackers (72).

■ Total calories: 402

Tropical Cottage Cheese: Have 170g (6oz) fat-free cottage cheese (180), 2 tbsp **sunflower seeds** (90), 115g (4oz) pineapple chunks tinned in juice (60) and 4 small wholemeal crackers (72).

■ Total calories: 402

Mediterranean Bean Roll-Ups: Warm 2 small corn tortillas (114) and spread with a mixture of 90g (3oz) rinsed and drained cannellini beans (150), 1 tbsp balsamic vinegar (5), 1 tsp olive oil (39), 1 tsp chopped fresh basil (0) and a shake of chilli powder (0). Top with 60g (2oz) sliced **avocado** (96) and 30g (1oz) shredded romaine lettuce (4).

■ Total calories: 408

Mini Pizzas: Spread 3 small corn tortillas (171) with 115g (4oz) passata (60), 10 large **black olives**, sliced (50), 30g (1oz) grated reduced-fat Cheddar cheese (80) and 90g (3oz) thinly sliced red pepper (24). Place under the grill or in the oven until the cheese begins to melt.

■ Total calories: 385

Monterey Jack Pitta Triangles: Slice 1 wholemeal pitta into quarters (140) and top with 2 tbsp salsa (9), 45g (1½oz) chopped red pepper (12), 45g (1½oz) chopped yellow pepper (12), 4 tbsp grated reduced-fat Monterey Jack cheese (81) and 10 large **black olives,** sliced (50). Place under the grill or in the oven to warm. Have with 1 medium apple (95).

◼ Total calories: 399

Olive and Mozzarella Sandwich: Sprinkle 2 slices wholemeal bread (160) with 10 large **black olives,** sliced (50), and 30g (1oz) grated reduced-fat mozzarella cheese (70). Place under the grill or in the oven to warm, if desired. Have with 1 medium pear (103).

◼ Total calories: 383

Chocolate Strawberry Yogurt: Mix 230g (8oz) fat-free plain yogurt (120) with 45g (1½oz) **dark chocolate chips** (207) and 115g (4oz) sliced fresh or thawed frozen unsweetened strawberries (52).

◼ Total calories: 379

Sweet Surprise Cereal: Melt 45g (1½oz) **dark chocolate chips** in a medium bowl in the microwave for 40 to 50 seconds (207). Add 45g (1½oz) puffed wheat cereal (105) and 2 tbsp raisins (66); stir to blend and allow to cool before eating.

◼ Total calories: 378

7.

WHEN YOU'RE OUT AND ABOUT

The Quick-and-Easy Meals and Snack Packs in this plan make it easy for you to follow the *Flat Belly Diet* rules when you have the time to plan ahead and make your meals. But what about those times when you're travelling, out running errands or stuck in the office and you forgot to bring your *Flat Belly Diet* meals? Look no further than this chapter to help you select the best choices to stick to your diet when you're out and about.

In this chapter, you'll find recommendations for choosing products which can provide a great shortcut for meals and snacks when you're short on time (see *Flat Belly Diet*-Friendly Products, opposite). You'll also find advice on making the best food choices when dining out and whenever you're stuck at the airport, in front of a vending machine, or in other spots where healthy eating may be a challenge (see Restaurant Rescue, opposite).

CAN A HOTEL BREAKFAST BE *FLAT BELLY DIET* FRIENDLY?

Over the past year, I've done a lot of travelling, and that means a lot of 'continental breakfasts'. Someone should start calling these 'Croissant Breakfasts' because these buttery pastries seem to be the tastiest things available. I've learned that eating healthily in hotels involves a lot of preparing ahead. To make your own *Flat Belly Diet* breakfast, pack small boxes of cereal, wholemeal crackers or packets of plain instant oatmeal as well as nuts or seeds (pre-measured in MUFA-size portions in individual zip-top bags), fruit packed in juice or water in individual serving cups and individual portions of shelf-stable milk, whether plain skimmed soya, almond, enriched rice or dairy milk.

FLAT BELLY DIET-FRIENDLY PRODUCTS

When shopping for your *Flat Belly Diet* feel free to choose the brands that are easily available to you and that fit your budget and location. Just keep in mind the MUFA Meal Maker Guidelines:

- Guideline #1: Consume no more than 4 grams of saturated fat per meal.
- Guideline #2: Ban trans fat.
- Guideline #3: Avoid artificial sweeteners, flavourings and preservatives.
- Guideline #4: Limit sodium to less than 2,300 milligrams a day.

As always, choose products with ingredients you can easily recognize and pronounce and foods (including frozen meals) that are made with whole grains, real produce, lean protein and low-fat dairy.

RESTAURANT RESCUE

Eating away from home is a part of everyday life for most people. Whether you're having a business lunch, meeting friends for dinner or taking the kids out for a special treat, I want you to be able to follow this plan. And it's easy to do. Here are a few key tips for staying on track when dining out.

- If you know in advance where you are going, check out the restaurant menu online. Find some meals that match your favourites in the meal plans. For those restaurants without a website, call in advance and ask for the menu to be faxed to you. Also, verify that the restaurant follows a trans-fat-free cooking policy, since trans fats must be eliminated on the *Flat Belly Diet*.

- At most restaurants, you can order a salad made of leafy greens (about the size of two tennis balls) topped with grilled chicken or salmon (about the size of a deck of cards) with balsamic or red wine vinegar and 2 tbsp of seeds or chopped nuts or 1 tbsp olive oil. Add a computer mouse-size serving of any one of the following: a wholemeal roll, baked or roasted potato, brown or wild rice or a starchy vegetable such as beans, peas or sweetcorn.

- Carry 2 tablespoons of nuts with you in a zip-top bag to supplement meals at restaurants where you might not be able to get a MUFA.

- Carry a tablespoon with you so that you can measure out nuts or seeds when they are provided by a restaurant.

The following pages offer guidance on ordering meals in different types of restaurants. The numbers in brackets are calorie amounts or ranges. MUFAs are listed in boldface. In some cases, you won't be able to find a MUFA in the menu, so bring along 2 tablespoons of nuts or seeds in a zip-top bag. A specific type of nuts or seeds that will complement your meal is listed, but feel free to substitute those that you have already packed or like best.

Different Types of Restaurants

A CHINESE RESTAURANT

Note: Chinese restaurants will let you order most dishes steamed. Most tea cups in a Chinese restaurant are about ½ cup, so you can use this to measure out your portions.

Order steamed mixed vegetables and have 2 cups (100). Have ½ cup steamed brown rice (if this is not available, select white rice) (80). Have 1 cup hot-and-sour soup or wonton soup (110). Order a side of **cashews** and measure out 2 tbsp (100); mix them with your vegetables and rice or have on the side.

Total calories: 390

Order 6 steamed vegetable dumplings (150). Have 1 cup steamed brown rice (if this is not available, select white rice) (160). Order a side of **cashews** and measure out 2 tbsp (100); sprinkle them over your vegetable dumplings and rice or have on the side.

Total calories: 410

Order steamed mixed vegetables with prawns and have 2 cups (200). Have 1/2 cup steamed brown rice (if this is not available, select white rice) (80). Order a side of **cashews** and measure out 2 tbsp (100); mix them with your vegetables and rice or have on the side.

Total calories: 380

THE DELI

Order a sandwich made of 2 slices wholemeal bread (160), 115g (4oz) organic sliced turkey (140), 3 tomato slices (5), a handful of shredded lettuce (0), 1 sachet of mustard (5) and 10 black or green **olives** (50). Have 1 medium apple (60).

Total calories: 420

Order 1 small salad (35), no dressing, with 6 tomato slices (10), 10 cucumber slices (10), 90g (3oz) grilled chicken (110) and a splash of balsamic vinegar (5). Order **olive oil** on the side and use your tablespoon to measure 1 tbsp (119). Have 1 slice wholemeal bread on the side (80).

Total calories: 369

AN ITALIAN TRATTORIA

Order cooked pasta, preferably wholewheat, and have a serving about the size of a tennis ball (175). Measure out 1 tbsp **olive oil** (119). Top your pasta with half of the oil plus 1 tbsp grated Parmesan cheese (22) and ground black pepper (0). Have a side salad (35); mix the other half of the oil with a splash of vinegar (5) to make a salad dressing. Have 180ml (6fl oz) (12 tbsp) minestrone soup (80) *or* a 60g (2oz) portion (the size of 2 matchbooks) of salmon that's baked or grilled with no added oil (90).

Total calories: 436–446

A JAPANESE SUSHI BAR

Note: Most tea cups in a Japanese restaurant are about ½ cup, so you can use this to measure out your portions. You can also use visual cues to stay on track; 1 cup steamed brown rice is about the size of a tennis ball.

Order tuna roll sushi and have 5 pieces (154). Have 1 cup steamed brown rice (if this is not available, select white rice) (160). Bring along 2 tbsp **cashews** (100).

Total calories: 414

Order cucumber roll sushi and have 6 pieces (136). Have 1 cup steamed brown rice (if this is not available, select white rice) (160). Bring along 2 tbsp **cashews** (100).

Total calories: 396

A PIZZERIA

Order 1 slice cheese pizza from a large pizza (272). Have a side salad (35) dressed with a splash of vinegar (5). Bring along 2 tbsp **pine nuts** (113).

Total calories: 425

A STEAKHOUSE

Order grilled steak and have 90g (3oz) (about the size of a deck of cards) (160). Have a serving of green beans, carrots or other vegetable about the size of a tennis ball (50) and ½ small baked potato (64). Order a side of **olive oil** and measure out 1 tbsp (119) to drizzle over the vegetables.

Total calories: 393

Order grilled chicken breast and have 90g (3oz) (about the size of a deck of cards) (160). Have a serving of green beans, carrots or other vegetable about the size of a tennis ball (50). Order a side of **olive oil** and measure out 1 tbsp (119) to drizzle over the vegetables. Have 1 small dinner roll, white or wholemeal (80).

Total calories: 409

Events and Entertainment Venues

Before you leave for the cinema, football match, carnival, theme park, or other destinations, pack your own *Flat Belly Diet* Snack Pack. Always include one small piece of fruit and 2 tablespoons of nuts or seeds packed in a zip-top bag. Also included here are some of the best choices you can make with what you might find available. The good news? Even these venues are beginning to offer healthier choices, including fresh fruit and nuts, thanks to demand from smart eaters like you!

A FOOTBALL MATCH

Have 60g (2oz), a small carton, caramel-coated popcorn (240). Bring 1 piece of fruit, like a small apple or medium orange (62), and 2 tbsp **peanuts** (110).

Total calories: 412

Have 1 small hamburger (254). Bring 1 piece of fruit, like a small apple or medium orange (62), and 2 tbsp **walnuts** (82).

Total calories: 398

Order a hot dog on a bun and have half (143) with 1 sachet of ketchup (15). Bring 1 piece of fruit, like a small apple or medium orange (62), and 2 tbsp **pumpkin seeds** (148).

Total calories: 368

Order corn tortilla chips and have about 16 chips (176). Bring 1 piece of fruit, like a small apple or medium orange (62), and 2 tbsp **peanuts** (110).

Total calories: 348

A CARNIVAL OR STREET FAIR

Order popcorn (air popped, without butter) and have 6 cups (about half of what you would find in a typical bag of microwave popcorn) (180). Bring 1 piece of fruit, like a small apple or medium orange (62), and 2 tbsp **peanuts** (110).

Total calories: 352

Order corn tortilla chips and have about 16 chips (176).
Bring 1 piece of fruit, like a small apple or medium orange
(62), and 2 tbsp **pumpkin seeds** (148).

Total calories: 386

THE CINEMA

Note: Consider taking along your snacks instead of buying food at
the cinema. You'll save money and stay the course with your diet.
Here are some *Flat Belly Diet*-approved suggestions.

Make Your Own Trail Mix 1: Combine 45g (1½oz) raisins (130),
2 tbsp **peanuts** (110) and 20 unsalted mini pretzels (110).

Total calories: 350

Make Your Own Trail Mix 2: Combine 45g (1½oz) **dark
chocolate chips** (207), 45g (1½oz) raisins (130) and 10
unsalted mini pretzels (55).

Total calories: 392

Bring 6 cups air-popped popcorn without butter (about
half of what you would find in a typical bag of microwave
popcorn) (180) and 45g (1½oz) **dark chocolate chips**
(207).

Total calories: 387

A THEME PARK

Order 1 small portion low-fat fudge ice cream (150). Bring 1 piece of fruit, like a small apple or medium orange (62), and 45g (1½oz) **dark chocolate chips** (207) to top your ice cream or to have on the side.

Total calories: 419

Order a hot dog on a bun and have half (143) with 1 sachet of ketchup (15). Bring 1 piece of fruit, like a small apple or medium orange (62), and 45g (1½oz) **dark chocolate chips** (207).

Total calories: 427

Order 1 slice cheese pizza (272) and 1 side salad (35) with a splash of vinegar (5). Bring along 2 tbsp **cashews** (100).

Total calories: 412

Order 1 small hamburger (254). Bring 1 piece of fruit, like a small apple or medium orange (62), and 2 tbsp **walnuts** (82).

Total calories: 398

A VENDING MACHINE

Get 2 oat and honey cereal bars (180). Bring 1 piece of fruit, like a small apple or medium orange (62), and 2 tbsp **pumpkin seeds** (148).

Total calories: 390

Get plain baked potato crisps, and have 60g (2oz) or 22 crisps (220). Bring 1 piece of fruit, like a small apple or medium orange (62), and 2 tbsp **peanuts** (110).

Total calories: 392

Get plain mini-crackers, and have 16 crackers (120) *or* get 100-calorie pack snacks (any variety with 3 grams or less saturated fat) (100). Bring 1 piece of fruit, like a small apple or medium orange (62), and 45g (1½oz) **dark chocolate chips** (207).

Total calories: 369–389

CONCLUSION

Losing belly fat helps your health but also gives you plenty of confidence. I know what it's like to work lots of hours and not find the time to shop for healthy foods, plan take-along meals and snacks and continue to eat healthily even while travelling. Celebrations, holidays and life can get in the way sometimes. But you can regain control over what you put in your mouth with this plan. Here you have the tools you need to follow the *Flat Belly Diet consistently* and make a flatter belly a reality.

Follow the *Flat Belly Diet* for as long as it takes for you to reach your goal weight. The 1,600-calorie plan was calculated to help you get to, and then also maintain, your goal weight. Diets shouldn't require a calorie readjustment for maintenance. The problem with most diets is that giving you fewer calories than it takes to support your healthy weight goal (then increasing once you get there) can cause not only a loss of body fat but also a loss of muscle mass and bone density, plus a weaker immune system. For most women, 1,600 calories provides enough calories to support your ideal or target weight – that means once you reach that weight, the plan will allow you to maintain it. If you continue to lose weight, beyond your goal weight, add back one-half to one snack until you begin to maintain your weight.

This plan is less about achieving a slim body than it is about creating a healthy life. The MUFAs and other healthful foods on the plan are just the fuel you need to fight disease and maintain your healthiest body ever.

COMMON CONVERSIONS

TEASPOON (TSP)	TABLESPOON (TBSP)	US CUPS	PINT	FLUID OUNCE (FL OZ)	MILLILITRE
1 tsp	1/3 tbsp				5ml
3 tsp	1 tbsp	1/16 cup		0.5fl oz	15ml
6 tsp	2 tbsp	1/8 cup		1fl oz	30ml
12 tsp	4 tbsp	1/4 cup		2fl oz	60ml
16 tsp	5 1/3 tbsp	1/3 cup		2.5fl oz	75ml
24 tsp	8 tbsp	1/2 cup		4fl oz	125ml
32 tsp	10 2/3 tbsp	2/3 cup		5fl oz	150ml
36 tsp	12 tbsp	3/4 cup		6fl oz	175ml
48 tsp	16 tbsp	1 cup		8fl oz	237ml
		2 cups		16fl oz	473ml
		3 cups	1 1/4 pints	24fl oz	710ml
		4 cups	1 3/4 pints	32fl oz	1 litres
		8 cups	3 1/2 pints	64fl oz	2 litres
		16 cups	7 pints	128fl oz	4 litres

YOUR MUFA SERVING CHART

FOOD	SERVING	CALORIES
OILS		
Flaxseed (linseed) oil (cold-pressed organic)	1 tbsp	120
Olive oil	1 tbsp	119
Peanut oil	1 tbsp	119
Pesto sauce	1 tbsp	80
Rapeseed oil	1 tbsp	124
Safflower oil (high oleic)	1 tbsp	120
Sesame or soya bean oil	1 tbsp	120
Sunflower oil (high oleic)	1 tbsp	120
Walnut oil	1 tbsp	120
NUTS, BEANS AND PULSES AND SEEDS		
Almonds	2 tbsp	109
Almond butter	2 tbsp	200
Brazil nuts	2 tbsp	110
Cashews	2 tbsp	100
Cashew butter	2 tbsp	190
Edamame (soya beans), shelled and boiled	230g (8oz)	298
Hazelnuts	2 tbsp	110
Macadamia nuts	2 tbsp	120
Peanuts	2 tbsp	110
Peanut butter (natural), crunchy	2 tbsp	188
Peanut butter (natural), smooth	2 tbsp	188

FOOD	SERVING	CALORIES
Pecans	2 tbsp	90
Pine nuts	2 tbsp	113
Pistachios	2 tbsp	88
Pumpkin seeds	2 tbsp	148
Sunflower seeds	2 tbsp	90
Sunflower seed butter	2 tbsp	190
Tahini (sesame seed paste)	2 tbsp	178
Walnuts	2 tbsp	82
AVOCADOS		
Avocado	60g (2oz)	96
OLIVES		
Black olive tapenade	2 tbsp	88
Green olive tapenade	2 tbsp	54
Green or black olives	10 large	50
DARK CHOCOLATE		
Dark chocolate chips	45g (1½oz)	207

EAT THESE FOODS REGULARLY
LEAN PROTEIN

FOOD	SERVING SIZE	CALORIES
BEANS AND PULSES		

Note: When using tinned beans, rinse in a colander for 2 to 3 minutes under cool running water to remove up to one-third of the sodium.

FOOD	SERVING SIZE	CALORIES
Adzuki beans, cooked	75g (2½oz)	147
Alfalfa sprouts	30g (1oz)	5
Baked beans, homemade with brown sugar	60g (2oz)	126
Baked beans, vegetarian	60g (2oz)	113
Baked beans, with beef or pork	60g (2oz)	113
Bean sprouts, kidney	30g (1oz)	30
Bean sprouts, mung	30g (1oz)	13
Black-eyed peas, cooked	75g (2½oz)	90
Black turtle beans, cooked	75g (2½oz)	120
Borlotti beans, cooked	75g (2½oz)	120
Broad beans, cooked	75g (2½oz)	62
Butter beans, cooked	90g (3oz)	105
Cannellini beans, cooked	75g (2½oz)	100
Chickpeas, cooked	75g (2½oz)	134
Chilli, vegetarian, canned	90g (3oz)	103
Chilli, with meat, low-fat, canned	90g (3oz)	154
Edamame (soya beans), unshelled, cooked	115g (4oz)	100
Green beans, cooked	115g (4oz)	114
Green beans, raw	90g (3oz)	30
Haricot beans, cooked	75g (2½oz)	104

FOOD	SERVING SIZE	CALORIES
Kidney beans, red, cooked	75g (2½oz)	110
Lentils, brown, cooked	115g (4oz)	115
Mung beans, cooked	75g (2½oz)	106
Pinto beans, cooked	75g (2½oz)	122
Refried beans, fat-free, tinned	90g (3oz)	45
Refried beans, traditional, tinned	90g (3oz)	100
Split peas, cooked	115g (4oz)	115
BEEF AND PORK		
Beef, chuck, lean, braised	90g (3oz)	179
Beef, topside, lean, roasted	90g (3oz)	138
Beef, fillet, lean	90g (3oz)	179
Beef, flank steak, lean	115g (4oz)	187
Beef, steak, sirloin, lean	90g (3oz)	166
Ham, low-sodium, 96% fat-free	30g (1oz)	31
Pork, chop, centre-cut, roasted	115g (4oz)	187
Pork fillet, roasted	90g (3oz)	115
EGGS		
Eggs	1 large	75
Egg white	60ml (2fl oz)	29

FOOD	SERVING SIZE	CALORIES
POULTRY		
Chicken breast, roasted	90g (3oz)	140
Chicken, drumstick, without skin, cooked	90g (3oz)	146
Chicken, minced, without skin, cooked	90g (3oz)	173
Chicken, thigh, boneless, without skin, cooked	90g (3oz)	166
Turkey burger, 90% lean, cooked	90g (3oz)	170
Turkey, organic slices	60g (2oz)	50
Turkey, drumstick, without skin, cooked	90g (3oz)	159
Turkey pepperoni, sliced	30g (1oz)	69
Turkey, roasted	90g (3oz)	162
Turkey sausage, Italian, lean, cooked	60g (2oz)	95
SEAFOOD		
Cod, Atlantic, baked	90g (3oz)	89
Crab, cooked	90g (3oz)	101
Crab, imitation (surimi)	90g (3oz)	87
Grouper, baked	90g (3oz)	100
Halibut, baked	90g (3oz)	119
Lobster, cooked	90g (3oz)	81
Plaice, baked	90g (3oz)	99
Pollack, baked or grilled	90g (3oz)	109
Prawns, grilled	115g (4oz)	120
Salmon, Alaskan, tinned	90g (3oz)	128
Salmon, wild, tinned, drained	90g (3oz)	135
Swordfish, baked	90g (3oz)	132
Tuna, chunks packed in water	90g (3oz)	120
Tuna, yellowfin, baked	90g (3oz)	118

FOOD	SERVING SIZE	CALORIES
DAIRY AND DAIRY ALTERNATIVES		
Cheddar cheese, reduced-fat, grated	60g (2oz)	81
Cottage cheese, fat-free	90g (3oz)	90
Feta cheese, crumbled	1 tbsp	40
Milk, skimmed	240ml (8fl oz)	80
Milk, 1% low-fat	240ml (8fl oz)	102
Parmesan cheese, grated	1 tbsp	21
Provolone cheese, reduced-fat	30g (1oz)	77
Rice milk, plain, enriched	240ml (8fl oz)	130
Ricotta cheese, fat-free	60g (2oz)	50
Sour cream, fat-free	1 tbsp	15
Soya milk, plain, unsweetened	240ml (8fl oz)	80
Yogurt, fat-free Greek-style	115g (4oz)	56
Yogurt, fat-free vanilla	115g (4oz)	103

FRUITS AND VEGETABLES

FOOD	SERVING SIZE	CALORIES
FRUIT		
Apple	1 medium	95
Apple sauce, unsweetened, tinned	90g (3oz)	33
Apricot	1 medium	17
Apricot, dried	6 pieces	60
Banana	1 small (6")	90
Blackberries	125g (4½oz)	62
Blueberries	60g (2oz)	40
Cantaloupe melon, balled	115g (4oz)	60
Cantaloupe melon, wedged	⅛ large	35
Cherries, sweet	60g (2oz)	50

FOOD	SERVING SIZE	CALORIES
Clementine	1 medium	40
Date, medjool, pitted	1 medium	66
Fig	1 large	47
Grapefruit	½ medium	60
Grapes, green or red	115g (4oz)	104
Guava	1 medium	61
Honeydew melon, balled	90g (3oz)	64
Honeydew melon, wedged	⅛ medium	58
Kiwi fruit (Chinese gooseberry), peeled	1 medium	46
Mandarin oranges, tinned	115g (4oz)	80
Mango, sliced	90g (3oz)	120
Nectarine	1 medium	70
Orange	1 medium	62
Papaya, cubed	90g (3oz)	55
Peach	1 medium	38
Pear	1 medium	104
Pineapple, sliced	90g (3oz)	100
Pineapple, chunks	115g (4oz)	60
Plum	1 (2")	30
Plum, sliced	60g (2oz)	47
Pomegranate	½ medium	53
Pomelo, sectioned	60g (2oz)	36
Raspberries	115g (4oz)	64
Rhubarb, diced	90g (3oz)	26
Star fruit (carambola)	1 medium	28
Tangerine	1 medium	50
Watermelon, chopped	90g (3oz)	45

FOOD	SERVING SIZE	CALORIES
VEGETABLES		
Artichoke	1 medium	60
Artichoke hearts, cooked, drained	90g (3oz)	42
Asparagus, cooked	125g (4½oz)	30
Aubergine, cubed, cooked, drained	230g (8oz)	35
Beetroot, cooked	90g (3oz)	37
Beetroot, pickled, whole, tinned	60g (2oz)	65
Broccoli, florets	150g (5½oz)	20
Brussels sprouts, cooked	115g (4oz)	65
Cabbage	¼ medium head	54
Carrot	1 medium	25
Carrots, cooked, drained	60g (2oz)	27
Cauliflower	¼ large head	53
Cauliflower, florets, cooked	150g (5½oz)	39
Celery	1 medium stalk	9
Celery, chopped	115g (4oz)	17
Courgette	1 medium	35
Courgette, sliced, steamed	115g (4oz)	25
Cucumber	1 (8")	45
Fennel bulb, sliced	115g (4oz)	27
Garlic	1 clove	4
Garlic, chopped	1 tsp	4
Ginger, fresh, grated	1 tbsp	5
Green beans, fresh	150g (5½oz)	35
Kale, curly, cooked	230g (8oz)	36
Lettuce, mixed baby	150g (4½oz)	15
Lettuce, romaine, chopped	60g (2oz)	8
Mushrooms, portobello	60g (2oz)	15
Mushrooms, portobello, grilled	90g (3oz)	29
Onion, chopped	60g (2oz)	34

FOOD	SERVING SIZE	CALORIES
Onion, red or yellow	1 medium	46
Onion, red or yellow, sliced	1 large slice	16
Pak choi, cooked, drained	125g (4½oz)	20
Pepper, ancho, dried	1 medium	47
Pepper, sliced	115g (4oz)	46
Rocket	115g (4oz)	28
Sauerkraut, low-sodium, canned	1 cup	31
Spring onion, top and bulb, chopped	30g (1oz)	16
Shallots, chopped	15g (½oz)	29
Spinach, baby	30g (1oz)	8
Spinach, cooked	90g (3oz)	41
Spring greens, chopped, cooked, drained	200g (7oz)	49
Swiss chard, chopped, cooked, drained	90g (3oz)	35
Tomato, plum	1 medium	12
Tomato, red	1 medium	35
Tomato, red, chopped	115g (4oz)	19
Tomato, red, pulped, tinned	125g (4½oz)	39
Tomato, red, sliced	1 slice	6
Tomatoes, cherry, red	150g (5½oz)	27
Tomato paste	1 tbsp	13

GRAINS AND STARCHY VEGETABLES

FOOD	SERVING SIZE	CALORIES
BREAD AND CRACKERS		
Bagel, wholemeal	30g (1oz)	75
Bread, French, wholemeal	1 slice (30g/1oz)	90
Bread, pitta, wholemeal	½ of 6" pita	70
Bread, wholemeal	1 slice (30g/1oz)	80
Breadcrumbs, dry	30g (1oz)	112
Bun, hamburger, wholemeal	1 bun (30g/1oz)	90
Cracker, crispbread, rye	20g (¾oz)	78
Cracker, small wholemeal	4 crackers	72
English muffin, wholemeal	60g (2½oz) or 1 muffin	140
Roll, dinner, wholemeal	1 roll (30g/1oz)	77
PASTA AND GRAINS		
Note: For most pasta shapes, 30g (1oz) of dry pasta makes approximately 170g (6oz) cooked.		
Barley, cooked	40g (1¼oz)	48
Bulgur, cooked	70g (2¼oz)	50
Crisps, baked	1 oz	120
Couscous, wholewheat, cooked	115g (4oz)	108
Oats, rolled, dry	60g (2oz)	150
Pasta or spaghetti, any shape, gluten-free, cooked	115g (4oz)	100
Pasta or spaghetti, any shape, wholewheat, cooked	115g (4oz)	87
Pilaf, 7-grain, cooked	60g (2oz)	85
Quinoa, cooked	60g (2oz)	81

FOOD	SERVING SIZE	CALORIES
Rice, basmati, cooked	110g (3½oz)	102
Rice, brown, medium grain, cooked	110g (3½oz)	109
Rice, wild, cooked	110g (3½oz)	83
Soba noodles, cooked	150g (5½oz)	113
Tortilla, corn	6"	57
Tortilla chips, multigrain, baked	15g (½oz)	60
STARCHY VEGETABLES		
Peas, cooked	60g (2oz)	62
Plantain	¼ medium	55
Potato, baked, with skin	1 medium	162
Potatoes, baby, roasted	150g (5½oz)	100
Potatoes, new, cooked	90g (3oz)	54
Squash, butternut, cubed, baked	200g (7oz)	82
Sweet potato, baked, without skin	1 medium	103
Sweet potato, cooked, mashed	115g (4oz)	125
Sweetcorn	1 large cob	123
Sweetcorn kernels	90g (3oz)	66

OTHER

FOOD	SERVING SIZE	CALORIES
SWEETENERS AND CONDIMENTS		
Apple butter	1 tbsp	29
Barbecue sauce	1 tbsp	12
Fruit spread, any flavour	1 tbsp	40
Honey	1 tsp	30
Horseradish sauce	1 tbsp	30
Ketchup	1 tbsp	16
Mayonnaise, rapeseed	1 tbsp	100
Mustard	1 tbsp	10

FOOD	SERVING SIZE	CALORIES
Mustard, Dijon, coarse-grain	1 tbsp	15
Salsa, medium	2 tbsp	9
Soy sauce	1 tbsp	11
Vinegar, balsamic or red wine	1 tbsp	10
Worcestershire sauce	1 tbsp	11
BEVERAGES		
Almond milk, unsweetened, original, vanilla or chocolate	240ml (8fl oz)	40–45
Cappuccino, with semi-skimmed milk	240ml (8fl oz)	73
Chai, with soya milk	240ml (8fl oz)	130
Coffee, iced latte, with skimmed milk	240ml (8fl oz)	47
Iced tea, unsweetened	240ml (8fl oz)	0
Tomato-vegetable juice, low-sodium	240ml (8fl oz)	53

If you don't like plain water, add any of the following juices once or twice per day to plain water for flavour. One fluid ounce of juice is 2 tablespoons. For the best results on the *Flat Belly Diet* plan, please account for the juice calories in your meal plan and please select 100 per cent juice only.

Apple juice	1fl oz	14
Cherry juice	1fl oz	19
Cranberry juice	1fl oz	17
Grape juice	1fl oz	19
Mango juice	1fl oz	18
Orange juice	1fl oz	14
Pineapple juice	1fl oz	16
Pomegranate juice	1fl oz	20

FOOD	SERVING SIZE	CALORIES
Prune juice	1fl oz	22
Tangerine juice	1fl oz	18

EAT THESE FOODS SPARINGLY

You can include these foods in your meals up to three times per week. For full-fat cheese, be sure to account for the saturated fat in your meal so you don't go over 4 grams of saturated fat per meal. Some full-fat cheeses have up to 6 grams of saturated fat per 30g (1oz) slice, so check your nutrition facts label.

FOOD	SERVING SIZE	CALORIES
PROTEIN		
Cheese, sliced, full-fat	30g (1 oz) or 1 slice	100–120
Cottage cheese, 2% reduced-fat	90g (3oz)	102
DAIRY		
Milk, 2% semi-skimmed	240ml (8fl oz)	122
GRAINS		
Bread or rolls, white flour	30g (1oz)	75
Crackers, white flour	15g (½oz)	61
Pasta, semolina, cooked	90g (3oz)	102
Pasta, white flour, cooked	90g (3oz)	95
Rice, white, cooked	110g (3½oz)	121
OTHER		
Sugar, granulated	1 tsp	16

INDEX

Bold page references indicate boxed text.